LACRIMAL DISORDERS
Diagnosis and Treatment

LACRIMAL DISORDERS
Diagnosis and Treatment

Everett R. Veirs, M.D.

Senior Consultant in Ophthalmology
Scott and White Clinic
Temple, Texas

with 183 illustrations

The C. V. Mosby Company

Saint Louis 1976

Printed in the United States of America

Distributed in Great Britain by Henry Kimpton, London

Library of Congress Cataloging in Publication Data

Veirs, Everett R 1908-
Lacrimal disorders.

Bibliography: p.
Includes index.
1. Lacrimal organs—Diseases. I. Title.
[DNLM: 1. Lacrimal apparatus diseases. 2. Lacrimal apparatus diseases—Congenital. WW208 V247La]
RE201.V39 617.7'64 76-16568
ISBN 0-8016-5233-2

CB/CB/B 9 8 7 6 5 4 3 2 1

This book is dedicated
to my wife,
Mary,
and my daughters,
Ann, Susan, and **Laura**

Preface

This monograph was written to present the information needed for a reasonable understanding of the lacrimal system, under both normal and abnormal conditions. The primary goal was to include material that would have the greatest practical value for the practicing ophthalmologist, the graduate student in ophthalmology, and to a lesser degree, the pediatrician and other physicians who often are the first to see patients with lacrimal disorders.

The techniques recommended for adequate examination and treatment of patients with lacrimal problems are for the most part those I have found to be the most satisfactory. This may make the treatise seem somewhat dogmatic, and to a degree that was intentional. Alternate methods are described in many instances, but to present many different techniques for most procedures could be confusing. The references were purposely kept brief and include only what was considered most important.

I am deeply indebted to a number of talented and dedicated people who helped in the preparation of this book. All contributed magnificently in their special fields. This list includes Miss Edrene Wallace, my hardworking and loyal secretary; Mr. Dave Hansen and his group in the Photographic Department; Mrs. Maribelle Mast, who prepared the fine drawings; and our institution's medical editor, Dr. Bernard K. Forscher. I am deeply indebted to Mrs. Billie Caughlin, who under Dr. Forscher's supervision did so many tasks in getting the manuscript ready.

Lastly, my greatest reward would be that this monograph result in physicians' taking greater interest in the many patients who have lacrimal disorders. Relieving these patients of their constant, nagging symptoms will bring gratification to the patient and a sense of satisfaction to the ophthalmologist.

Everett R. Veirs

Contents

CHAPTER 1

Anatomy and embryology of the lacrimal system

ANATOMY

The eyelids

The eyelids are made up of many structures essential to the proper comfort and function of the eye. Externally, the eyelids are covered with a delicate, thin skin that allows the lids to move freely when the eyelids open and close, while at the same time a lesser movement occurs in a horizontal direction. The subcutaneous tissue, orbicularis oculi muscle, and areolar tissue are external to the tarsi, which is tough, dense, fibrous tissue. The tarsi, extending from the puncta laterally for a distance of 25 to 30 mm, give body and shape to the lids. The upper tarsus has its convexity superiorly and its greatest height at the middle of the lids, a fact easily observed in doing levator surgery. A thin, fibrous layer extends from the tarsi to the septum orbitale to the periosteum of the orbital margin and to the medial and lateral palpebral tendons.

Horizontal folds mark the level of the upper border of the tarsus in the upper lid and the lower border of the tarsus in the lower lid. The aponeurosis of the levator palpebrae superioris passes between the upper orbital margin and the eye, its upper margin fusing with the septum orbitale superior to the tarsus. The central portion of the aponeurosis of the levator is attached to the skin of the lid and the anterior surface of the tarsus in its lower 4 mm or so. The fascia sheaths of the levator muscle form an attachment with the sheath of the superior rectus muscle. Numerous glands empty on the conjunctival side of the lids as well as at the lid margin (Fig. 1-1).

The orbicularis oculi muscle consists of the orbital part and the palpebral part. The palpebral part originates from (1) the medial palpebral tendon, (2) the deep fascia that covers the upper portion of the lacrimal sac, and (3) the posterior lacrimal crest (Horner's or tensor tarsi or pars lacrimalis is the pretarsal portion of the muscle) (Fig. 1-2). The tensor tarsi muscle runs forward and laterally to insert in the connective tissue surrounding the canaliculi and the medial part of the tarsal plates.

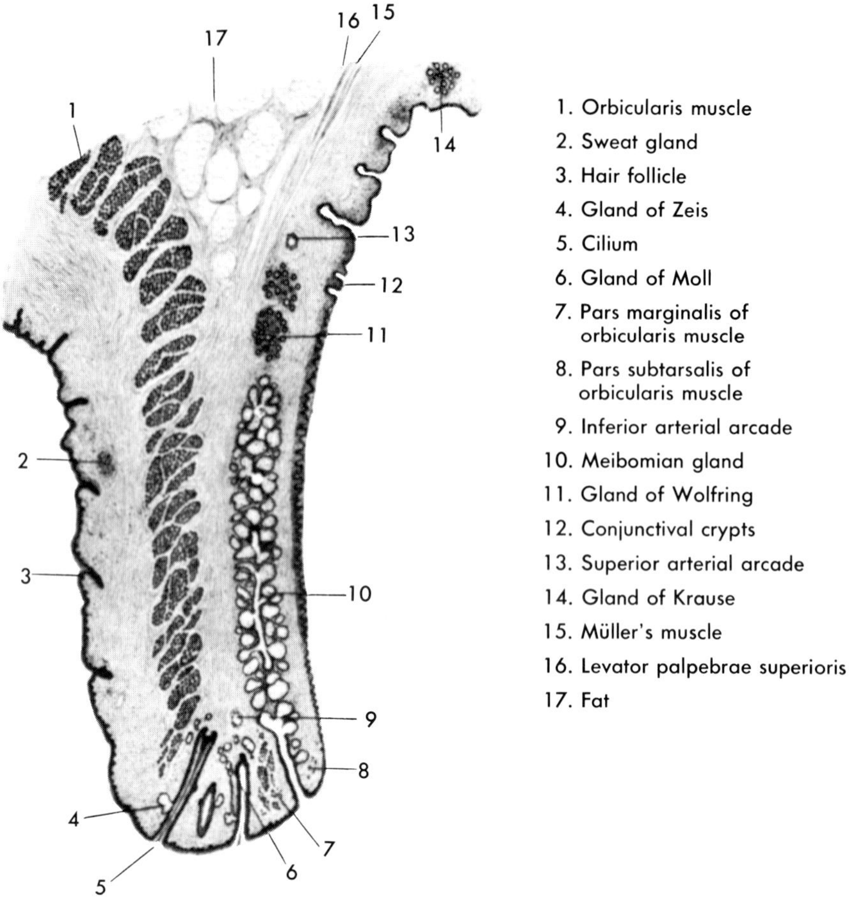

Fig. 1-1. Structure of eyelid. (From Duke-Elder, S.: System of ophthalmology, vol. II, St. Louis, 1961, The C. V. Mosby Co., p. 506.)

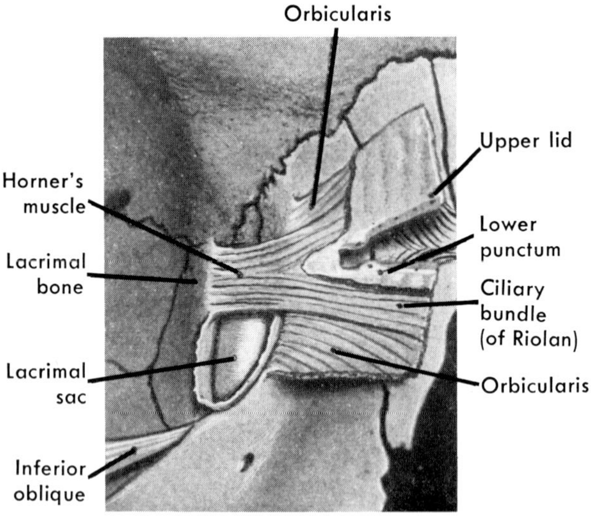

Fig. 1-2. Lid retracted medially to show origin and insertion of Horner's muscle and origin of orbicularis oculi muscles. (From Last, R. J.: Wolff's anatomy of the eye and orbit, ed. 5, Philadelphia, 1961, W. B. Saunders Company, p. 205.)

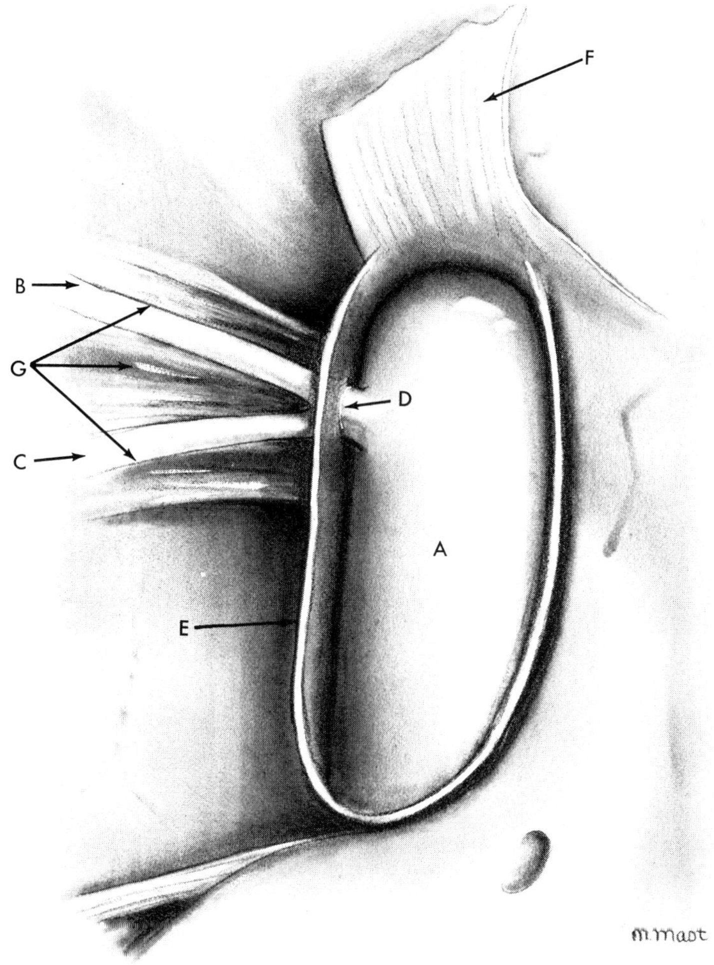

Fig. 1-3. *A,* Lacrimal sac; *B,* upper canaliculus; *C,* lower canaliculus; *D,* common canaliculus passing through lacrimal fascia; *E,* lacrimal fascia; *F,* medial palpebral tendon (reflected up) continuous with lacrimal fascia posteriorly; *G,* Horner's muscle running forward to insert into tissue surrounding canaliculi and tarsal plate medially. (Redrawn after Last, R. J.: Wolff's anatomy of the eye and orbit, ed. 5, Philadelphia, 1961, W. B. Saunders Company.

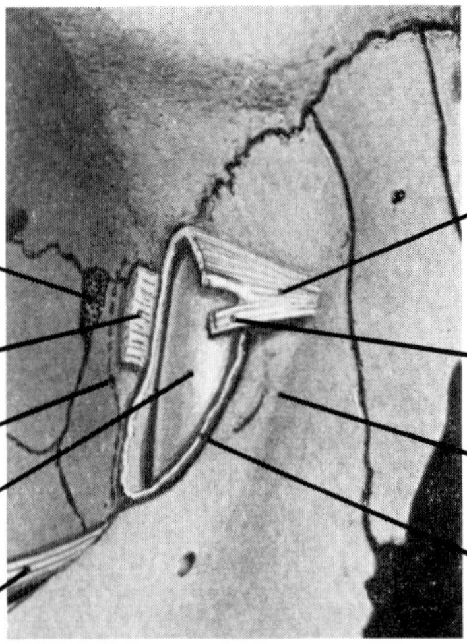

Fig. 1-4. Lacrimal fascia (periorbita) enclosing the lacrimal sac (fascia anterior to sac cut away to show sac). Upper border of medial palpebral tendon blends with tough periorbita that is strongly attached to bone just superior to dome of sac. Acute dacryocystitis will cause swelling only inferior to medial palpebral tendon. If swelling occurs superiorly to tendon, tumor is highly probable. (From Last, R. J.: Wolff's anatomy of the eye and orbit, ed. 5, Philadelphia, 1961, W. B. Saunders Company, p. 206.)

The tensor tarsi muscles are important in helping to keep the lids in proper position to function. The muscle has its origin more posteriorly than the origin of the remainder of the orbicularis oculi muscles. As the muscle passes laterally toward its insertion, it splits so that the portion to the upper lid passes upward and outward, and the portion to the lower lid passes downward and outward (Figs. 1-2 and 1-3). Also, the origin of this muscle is centered so as to have the greatest direct medial pull during contraction (Fig. 1-3). The muscle probably is mainly responsible for keeping the puncta turned backward to be in proper contact with the eyeball and for assisting in the movement medially of the puncta and their closure with lid contraction.

The position of the medial palpebral ligament (tendon) is of great importance in lacrimal surgery (Fig. 1-4). The ligament takes its origin from an extensive area of the frontal process of the maxilla beginning at this anterior lacrimal crest and extending anteriorly to about the nasomaxillary suture. There is no advantage in severing the medial palpebral tendon in performing a routine external dacryocystorhinostomy. Because the common canaliculus empties into the lacrimal sac posterior to this tendon, severing the tendon may be indicated in rare cases. In operations to bring the dome of the sac into the lacrimal lake region (Stallard procedure to reestablish tear drainage in the absence of patent canaliculi), the tendon must be severed. If the tendon is severed, it should be resutured with a permanent type of strong suture. The reason that

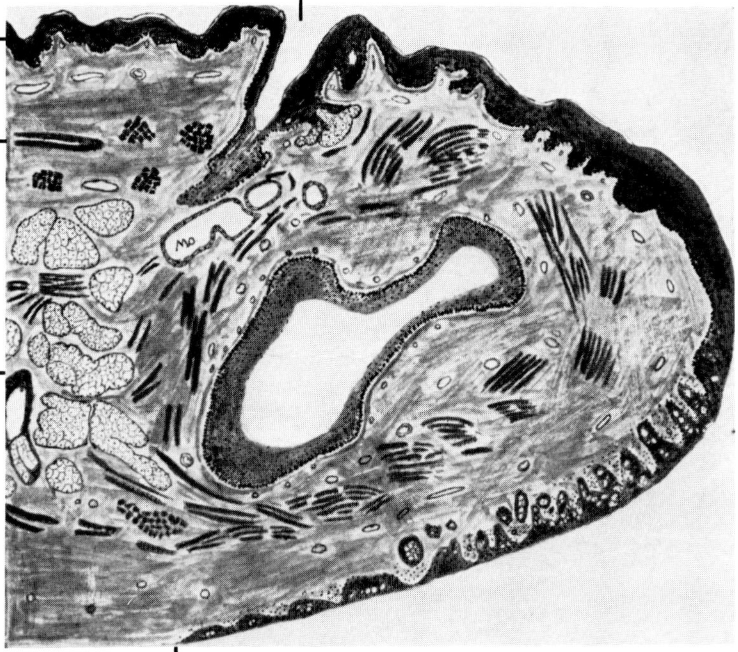

Fig. 1-5. Cross section of medial portion of lower lid demonstrating lacrimal canaliculus at junction of horizontal and vertical portions surrounded by fibers of orbicularis and lying in bed rich in elastic tissue. Canaliculi are lined by stratified squamous epithelium. (From Last, R. J.: Wolff's anatomy of the eye and orbit, ed. 5, Philadelphia, 1961, W. B. Saunders Company, p. 204.)

lateral lid retraction does not occur more often when the tendon is severed is that the tendon has such an extensive origin, especially from the deep fascia that covers the upper part of the sac.

The canaliculi

The vertical part of the canaliculi is 2 to 2.5 mm long and begins at the lacrimal punctum. The diameter of the punctum is about 0.2 to 0.3 mm, approximately half that of the canaliculus. The horizontal portion of the canaliculus is 7 to 8 mm long from the punctum to the inner canthus; the upper part is slightly shorter than the lower. Each canaliculus may pierce the lacrimal fascia separately before joining to form the common canaliculus (sinus of Maier). In some instances the canaliculi join before piercing the lacrimal fascia. Narrowing may occur in the canaliculi where they traverse the fascia. The region where the common canaliculus empties into the lacrimal sac is termed "the ampullary portion of the common canaliculus" and is a common site of stenosis. This site is at the midpoint of the medial palpebral tendon and slightly posterior to the midlateral surface of the sac. The canaliculi have elastic walls, allowing them to be stretched in any direction and also allowing their lumen to be dilated to two or three times their normal (0.5 mm) diameter (Fig. 1-5). Unfortunately, great harm can result from traumatic dilatation of the canaliculus. Not infrequently, beginning about in middle age, the lumen of the canaliculi will narrow, especially that portion closest to the lacrimal sac. Trauma in probing easily converts a partial stenosis to a complete closure, with an increase in severity of symptoms.

The lacrimal sac

The lacrimal fossa containing the lacrimal sac is easily located because it is in the anteromedial wall of the orbit. The medial palpebral tendon is a key landmark, just anterior to the upper few millimeters of the sac. The sac is enclosed by the lacrimal fascia (periorbita) except for the lower 3 to 4 mm of the sac. This periorbita is strongly attached to the anterior lacrimal crest from which it splits into two layers that enclose the sac and then join and attach tightly to the posterior lacrimal crest. In performing operations on the lacrimal sac, it is wise to make the vertical incision beginning 2 to 4 mm medially and just below the medial palpebral tendon. The incision should be carried nearly vertically, curving only a little laterally, and should include the periosteum. Because the angular vessels are curved (concavity outward), these vessels or larger branches will be cut with most incisions, but this is of no real importance (Fig. 1-6). The periosteum that was cut with the original incision is tightly bound to the bone, and a sharp periosteal elevator is required (sharp-bladed Freer elevator is satisfactory) to separate the periosteum laterally to the anterior lacrimal crest. Pressing the elevator slightly against the bone at the anterior lacrimal crest and separating the periosteum in a vertical direction along the crest will possibly decrease the chances of injuring the lacrimal sac.

The lacrimal periosteum is easily separated from the bone posterior to the crest, so the sac can be retracted laterally without difficulty as the operation proceeds.

The strong attachment of the lacrimal fascia to the posterior lacrimal crest is a protective barrier against exposing orbital fat. This seldom happens because the posterior crest is far back and is seldom disturbed. The thickness of the bone of the frontal process of the maxilla varies enormously. Much of this bone must be removed to allow for an anastomosis of adequate size to be made into the nose. The mucous membrane of the nose is seen as soon as an opening is made in this bone. For most operations the bone medial to the anterior lacrimal crest should be removed first (Fig. 1-7). As the bony opening is enlarged, the posterior part becomes thinner to the point where the bone separating the nasal mucosa and lacrimal sac mucosa is paper thin in most instances.

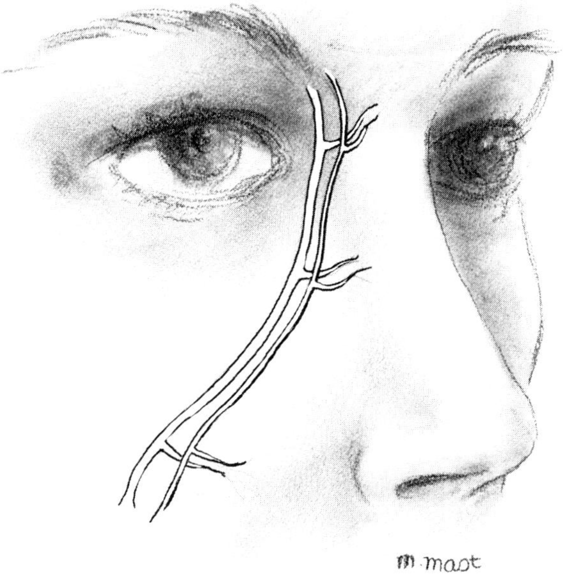

Fig. 1-6. Approximate course of vessels (vein is nearer to eye). Incision of one or more vessels is difficult to avoid when operating on lacrimal sac unless incision is made far nasally. With proper technique, incised vessels are usually easily handled (see Chapter 11).

Although the lacrimal fossa with the lacrimal sac is about 14 mm long, the upper 5 mm or so of the sac (all of the sac above the lower border of the medial palpebral tendon) should not be disturbed unless an unusual pathologic process exists superiorly. Extending the anastomosis to that height would disturb ethmoid cells and would damage vital structures as well (Fig. 1-8).

The lacrimal sac is continuous with the nasolacrimal duct which, as it passes downward, veers slightly outward and backward and is encased in bone for about 12 mm (Fig. 1-9). The nasolacrimal duct empties into the nose beneath the inferior turbinate; its last 3 to 5 mm is surrounded by soft tissues.

Often, a sufficiently large anastomosis from the lacrimal sac into the nose is not obtained by removing only the bone from the lower border of the medial palpebral tendon to the upper border of the nasolacrimal duct. Obtaining the proper size and proper position of the anastomosis requires not only removing bone as far as the lower edge of the lacrimal crest but also removing bone along this line for another 3 to 4 mm inferiorly. After this bone is removed, it is usually a simple matter to use a straight bone-biting forceps to remove the rather thin bone that separates the upper 3 to 4 mm of the nasolacrimal duct mem-

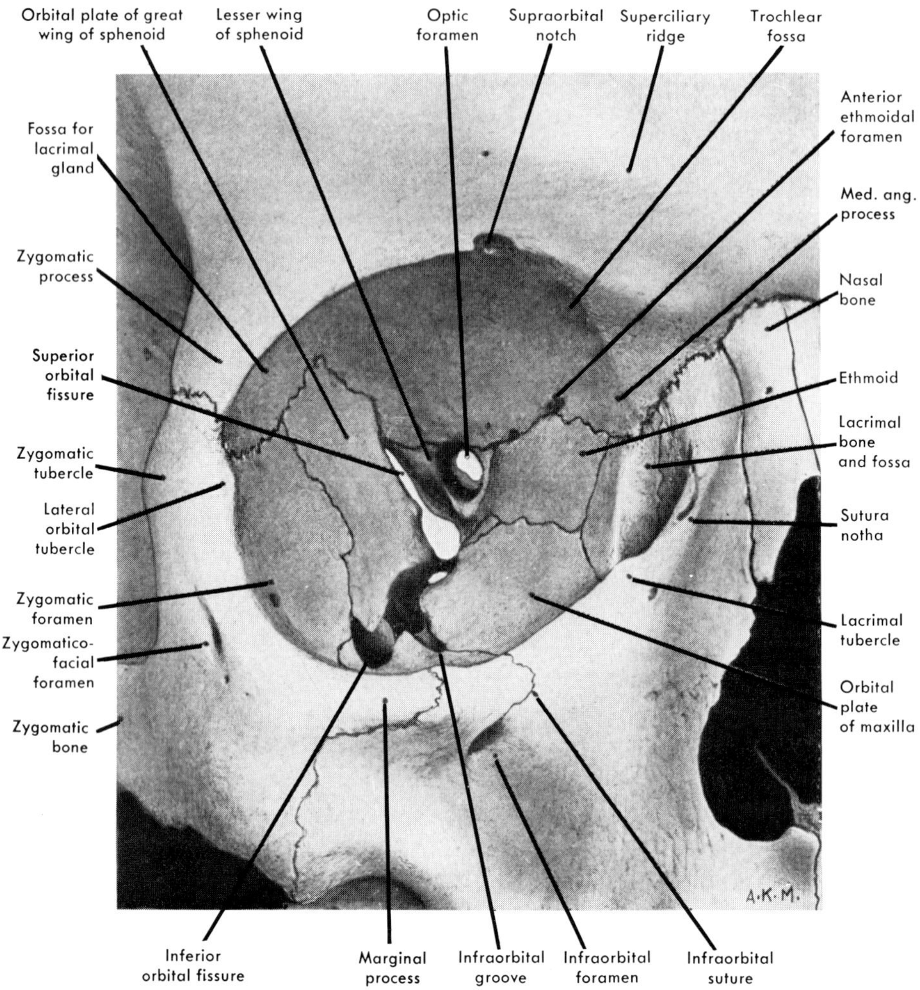

Fig. 1-7. Orbit as viewed from front. (From Last, R. J.: Wolff's anatomy of the eye and orbit, ed. 5, Philadelphia, 1961, W. B. Saunders Company, p. 3.)

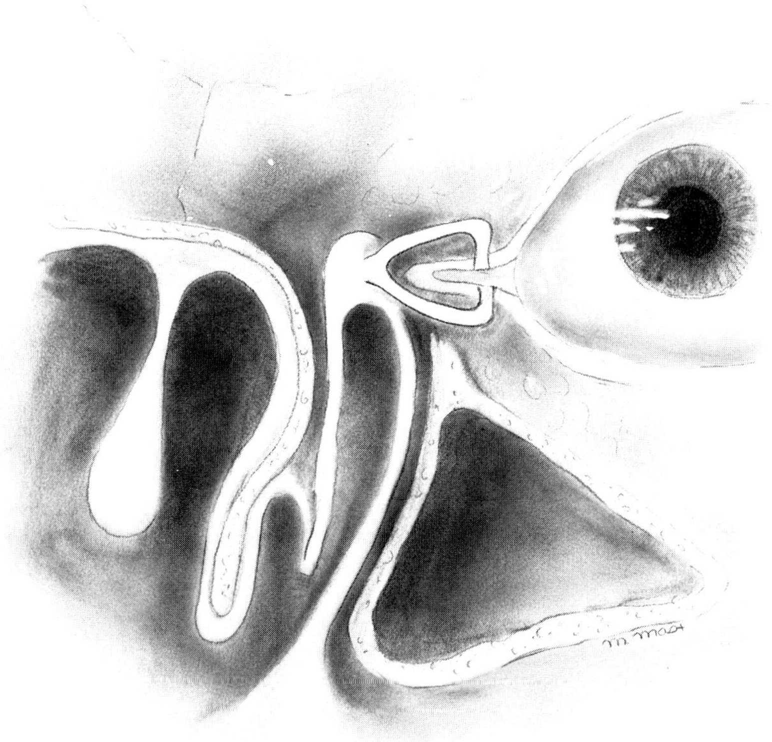

Fig. 1-8. Lacrimal drainage system. Lacrimal sac shown here is as it would appear with some pathologic problem (for example, dacryocystitis or tumor). Normally it is little more than a potential space.

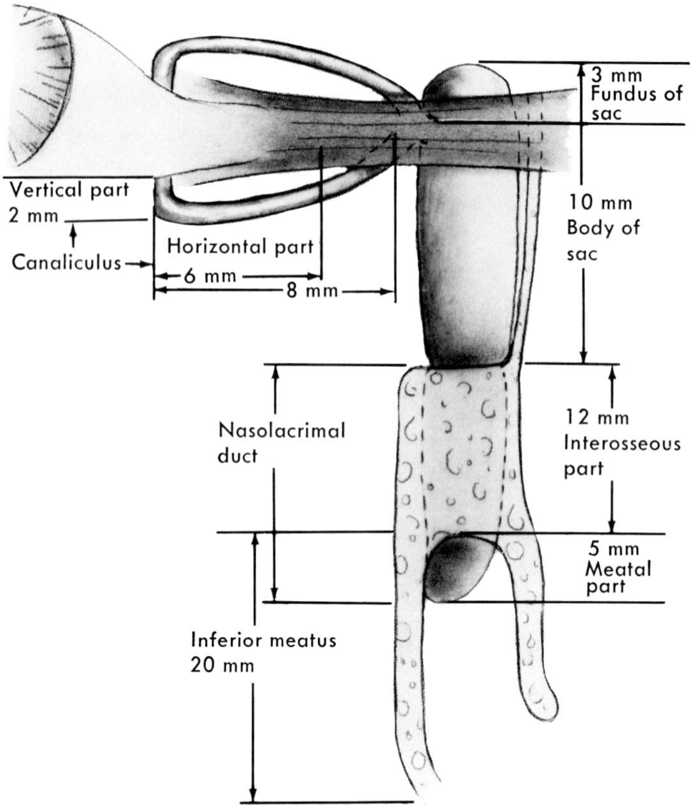

Fig. 1-9. Approximate measurements of lacrimal drainage channels. (Modified from Jones, L. T., Reeh, M. J., and Wirtschafter, J. D.: Ophthalmic anatomy, p. 70. By permission of American Academy of Ophthalmology and Otolaryngology, Rochester, Minn. 1970.)

brane and the nasal mucosa, allowing for a much larger anastomosis in an area free from obstruction.

The antrum can be entered unintentionally if the bone is removed too far laterally after the operator has reached the lower end of the anterior lacrimal crest. This is more likely in young patients, especially if the original incision is curved too laterally. The error is easily recognized because the sinus mucosa is much thinner than the nasal mucosa.

EMBRYOLOGY

Development anomalies of the lacrimal system are easily understood if the basic embryology of the system is clear.

The drainage passages

The drainage passages account for the vast majority of these anomalies. Early in embryonic development, a solid column of ectodermal cells becomes

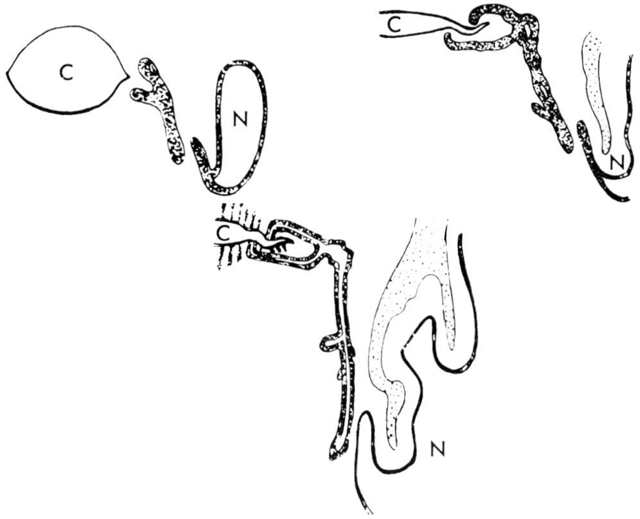

Fig. 1-10. *Upper left,* At 6 weeks' gestation. Solid column of ectodermal cells has become buried in mesoderm. Two short columns budding off main body superiorly represent anlages of upper and lower canaliculi. Second rod of epithelial cells apparently is developing from nasal cavity to join larger, more superior column of cells. *C,* Conjunctival sac; *N,* nasal cavity. *Upper right,* At 12 weeks' gestation. Lysis of column of cells has begun. Anlages of canaliculi have reached lid margin. *Bottom,* At 14 weeks' gestation. Lysis has produced patent channel except inferiorly. Opening of lower end of nasolacrimal duct into nose normally occurs just before or just after birth. (From Duke-Elder, S., and Cook, C.: The lids, conjunctiva and lacrimal apparatus. The lid folds. In System of ophthalmology, vol. III, St. Louis, 1963, The C. V. Mosby Co., p. 242.)

buried in the cleft between the maxillary process and the lateral nasal process. As the maxillary process develops further and fuses with the lateral nasal process, the solid column of ectodermal cells becomes buried, surrounded by mesoderm. The lacrimal canaliculi develop when the upper extremity of the epithelial cells bifurcate in the developing inner canthal region. By the third month the column of cells that forms the canaliculi has reached the lid margins, and the cells that will form the lacrimal region will have proliferated and begun to degenerate to form cavities. The process of disintegration of the column of epithelial cells continues downward from the dome of the primitive sac (Fig. 1-10).

According to Leplat,[1] a second rod of epithelial cells appears to emerge from the developing nasal cavity and to elongate upward, laterally to the inferior turbinate, to lie adjacent to the lower end of the nasolacrimal duct. Lysis of the central cells at the point of junction of the two columns of cells, usually at about 6 months' gestation, completes the tear drainage channel, which extends from the punctum into the nose.

The most common congenital anomaly of the system, occlusion of the nasolacrimal duct, probably can be explained on the basis of the two rods of epithelial cells having to join to form one lumen after degeneration of their central cells; in the rare infant who seems to have an osseous occlusion instead of a membranous one, perhaps the two columns failed to join.

The lacrimal glands

The lacrimal glands include a number of glands that are widely dispersed, vary in histologic structure, and most importantly, vary in the nature of their secretions. Disorders involving the system can vary from the mild and transient to the severe.

The lacrimal gland stems from the conjunctival lining of basal cells in the outer upper fornix. Several solid columns of cells move upward and become surrounded by mesoderm. These solid columns increase in number and size and finally develop into ducts. The secretory elements of the gland are derived from mesoderm.

REFERENCE

1. Cited by Duke-Elder, S., and Cook, C.: The ocular adnexa. In System of ophthalmology, vol. XIII, St. Louis, 1974, The C. V. Mosby Co., pp. 231-246.

CHAPTER 2

Physiology of the lacrimal system

Normal secretion and drainage of tears is essential for the proper functioning and comfort of the eye. Although a great deal is known about the anatomy of the lacrimal system, the secretion of tears, the physical and chemical properties of tears, and the drainage mechanism, many questions remain unanswered. A knowledge of the basic principles of the functioning of the lacrimal system is often essential for the proper diagnosis and treatment of its disorders.

SOURCES OF TEARS

The lacrimal fluid is made up of the watery secretions of the main lacrimal gland and of the accessory glands of Krause and Wolfring, all serous glands. The main lacrimal gland is divided into two lobes, the larger orbital lobe that lies in the lacrimal fossa just posterior to the outer bony orbital rim and the palpebral lobe that lies anterior and inferior to the orbital lobe. The two lobes are separated by the lateral extension of the aponeurosis of the levator muscle. (It has been suggested[8] that the orbital lobe be called the main lacrimal gland and the palpebral lobe, the accessory palpebral gland.) The ducts of the orbital lobe traverse the palpebral lobe and, together with the ducts of the palpebral lobe, empty into the conjunctival sac just in front of the upper fornix in its outer half. However, one or more ducts may empty below the lateral canthus. Removal of the palpebral gland theoretically should prevent tears from the orbital lobe and the palpebral lobe from reaching the conjunctival sac.

The palpebral lobe of the lacrimal gland often may be easily visualized, especially in prominent eyes, by everting the lid or by pulling the temporal portion of the upper lid outward and upward. Occasionally, a dermolipoma may be mistaken for this portion of the gland.

The accessory glands of Krause and of Wolfring are situated subconjunctivally, chiefly above the upper tarsus; a few are inferior to the lower tarsus. The glands of Krause are more numerous and are located at the fornix. The glands of Wolfring are near the tarsal margin.

The oil glands empty at the lid margins and consist of (1) the meibomian glands, about 20 on each lid and by far the most important of the oil glands, (2) the glands of Zeis, which are accessory sebaceous glands, and (3) the glands of Moll, located at the eyelash roots. The goblet cells that secrete the mucin are widely scattered in the conjunctiva, chiefly the palpebral conjunctiva.

NERVE SUPPLY

The lacrimal gland is innervated by (1) the lacrimal nerve, a branch of cranial nerve V, which is believed to be the afferent path of the reflex arc and (2) the facial parasympathetic nerve, which originates in the pons, joins the facial nerve, passes through the facial nucleus and geniculate ganglion, and joins the great superficial petrosal nerve. The sympathetic fibers from the internal carotid plexus join the superficial petrosal nerve to form the vidian nerve (nerve of the pterygoid canal), which ends in the sphenopalatine ganglion where the parasympathetic fibers synapse. The parasympathetic fibers join the zygomatic branch of the maxillary division of nerve V until it branches off to join the lacrimal nerve just posterior to the orbital lobe of the lacrimal gland. In addition to the sympathetic fibers accompanying the parasympathetic ones, some fibers reach the gland by accompanying the lacrimal artery. Studies in cats[2] suggest that the stimulation for the secretion of tears originates in or passes through the sphenopalatine ganglion but not through the superior cervical ganglion and does not activate secretory cells of the lacrimal gland. Thus, the parasympathetic fibers, and not the sympathetic fibers, are responsible for carrying the impulses that result in lacrimal gland secretion.

THE PRECORNEAL FILM

The precorneal film consists of three layers: (1) the inner or mucoid layer that rests against the corneal epithelium in a thin sheet and that contains mucins or high-molecular-weight glycoproteins that act as a natural wetting agent for the eye; (2) the middle (the thickest) layer, a watery fluid secreted by the lacrimal glands; and (3) the outer layer, an oily one.

PHYSIOLOGY OF TEAR SECRETION

The secretion of tears is a continuous process and is maintained by the accessory lacrimal glands, the glands that produce mucin and oil, and the main lacrimal gland. Most authorities agree that the reflex lacrimal secretion of tears is the exclusive function of the main lacrimal gland. Also, most authorities agree that the efferent parasympathetic nerves carry stimulation to the main glands. Duke-Elder[3] and Whitwell[16] believe that the sympathetic system is responsible for reflex excess secretion. It is possible to maintain an adequate tear film with the accessory glands plus the mucin- and oil-producing glands, as demonstrated by removal of the main lacrimal gland. However, removal of the main gland will occasionally result in an inadequate amount of tear secretion.

Reflex stimulation of excess tear secretion may result from irritative stimuli of any of the divisions of cranial nerve V but is more pronounced with stimulation of the ophthalmic division. Disease and injuries of the cornea and irritation of the nasal mucosa are classic examples of reflex stimulation.

Function of tears

The precorneal films serve many essential functions such as helping keep the cornea uniformly smooth for the best optical results and for comfort, preventing irritation of the cornea from drying and by mechanically removing foreign matter, and aiding in the metabolism of the cornea. The tears contain an enzyme (lysozyme) and immunoglobulins, both of which have antibacterial qualities. The content of lysozyme in tears may be decreased in various situations. For example, patients with eye irritation due to smog were found to have a tear lysozyme content averaging 60% less than mean normal levels.[14] Decreased tear lysozyme content also is found in such disorders as keratoconjunctivitis sicca, trachoma, and chronic cicatricial conjunctivitis (ocular pemphigus).

Tears not only lubricate the cornea but also lubricate the opposing surfaces of the conjunctiva (bulbar and palpebral conjunctivae) with the movements of the lids and eyes. The oil film on the lid margins aids in preventing the overflow of tears onto the skin.[1] The majority of full-term and some premature newborn babies have been found to secrete tears during their first 24 hours of life.

Quantity of tear secretion

Under normal conditions it is estimated that the average person secretes about 1 g of tears during a 24-hour period, mostly during the waking hours. This can vary considerably, and on the average the amount is considerably more in the young than in the elderly.

MEASUREMENT OF TEAR FORMATION

Schirmer test

This test, using Whatman No. 41 filter paper cut into strips 5 by 30 mm, is a valuable but often ignored clinical method for measuring the amount of tear secretion. The strip is folded 5 mm from one end, and this short segment is placed into the conjunctival sac at the junction of the outer one third and the inner two thirds of the lower lid. However, it is just as satisfactory to place the folded strip on the inner aspect of the lower lid. The patient should be instructed to look upward while the Schirmer test is being performed (see Fig. 3-1).

Most healthy eyes in the relatively young will show moistening of about 15 mm of the exposed portion of the paper. The elderly may be symptomless with no more than 5 mm of wetting (histologic examination shows atrophy of the lacrimal gland with or without increased collagenous and adipose tissue). There is a progressive diminution of tear formation with age until in the sixth and seventh decades the lacrimation is only one third to one fourth that of the first two decades.[15] Hypersecretors may show 25 mm of moistening in 1 minute or less.

An apparent marked increase in tear secretion as measured by the Schirmer test may be due to obstruction of the lacrimal drainage system. This can be easily demonstrated by performing the Schirmer test bilaterally on a patient who has obstruction on one side only.

It is recognized that insertion of the filter paper to measure the amount of tear secretion causes some irritation of the eye and therefore some reflex secretion, but this can be abolished by instilling a topical anesthetic several minutes before the test is performed. From a practical point of view this and other variations of the test (such as measuring the amount of tear formation by stimulating the nasal mucosa with wisps of cotton or fumes such as those from ammonia) seldom give much helpful information. The use of a phenol red paper strip, a pH indicator, has been recommended[6] as more suitable than Whatman filter paper in performing the Schirmer test.

Dye dilution

The use of a lacrimal streak dilution test is recommended by Norm[13]; in this test the amount of dye (fluorescein and rose bengal mixture) is used to evaluate tear secretion. After the dye is instilled into the conjunctival sac, an intense red color is observed in the streak of tears collecting at the lower lid margin. The dilution of the dye by the tears is observed through a slitlamp, and the color is compared to a color scale. With normal tear formation the streak is quickly diluted to a pale yellow. With a scanty amount of tears the red streak will persist after 5 minutes have passed. By this technique of measurement, production has been shown to range from 15 to 30 g in a 24-hour-period, far greater than the value of 1 g usually stated. The discrepancy is due to the fact that in the Schirmer test by far the greatest amount of tears escapes through the nasolacrimal duct. With measurement of the amount of tear formation by the lacrimal streak dilution method it is possible to determine concomitantly if there is staining of the cornea (as seen in keratoconjunctivitis sicca) and patency of the nasolacrimal system.

CHARACTERISTICS OF TEARS

Table 1 compares tears to plasma in regard to a number of components and properties.

Osmotic pressure

The osmotic pressure, expressed as equivalent to grams of NaCl per 100 g of water, averages about 0.9. Studies[9] of persons with normal eyes[9] showed a range of 0.903 to 0.950, with the total osmotic pressure of tears of patients with various pathologic conditions of the eye usually falling within this range. These studies demonstrated that after instillation of 0.2 ml of 2.5% saline into

Table 1. Properties and components of human tears and plasma*

	Tears	*Plasma*
Properties		
Osmotic pressure	Equiv 0.9% NaCl	6.62 atm
pH	7.4 (7.3 to 7.7)	7.39
Refractive index	1.357	1.35
Solids		
Water content (g/100 ml)	98.2	94.0
Ash (g/100 ml)	1.05	0.6 to 1.0
Total solids (g/100 ml)	1.8	8.6
Electrolytes		
Bicarbonate (meq/liter)	26	24.3
Chloride (meq/liter)	135	102
Potassium (meq/liter)	15 to 29	5
Sodium (meq/liter)	142	137 to 142
Nitrogen compounds		
Total protein (g/100 ml)	0.669 to 0.800	6.7
Albumin (g/100 ml)	0.394	4.0 to 4.8
Globulin (g/100 ml)	0.275	2.3
Ammonia (mg/100 ml)	5	0.047
Urea (mg/100 ml)	40	26.8
Total nitrogen (g/100 ml)	0.158	1.114
Nonprotein nitrogen (mg/100 ml)	51	15 to 42
Carbohydrate		
Glucose (mg/100 ml)†	0 to 5.0	80 to 90
Other		
Citric acid (mg/100 ml)	0.6	2.2 to 2.8
Ascorbic acid (mg/100 ml)	0.14	0.1 to 0.7

*Modified from Milder, B.: The lacrimal apparatus. In Moses, R. A., editor: Adler's physiology of the eye, clinical application, ed. 6, St. Louis, 1975, The C. V. Mosby Co., pp. 17-34.
†Because of the close correlation between the glucose content of the tears and that of the blood, the glucose content of the tears will increase sufficiently to give a positive reaction with the paper test strip (Clinistix) in about 85% of patients with a blood sugar value of 160 mg/100 ml or above.

the conjunctival sac the saline was diluted to the concentration of normal tears within two minutes. The osmotic pressure of tears is the same as that of the aqueous humor and of blood plasma.

Hydrogen ion concentration

The pH of tears varies not only among different persons but also at different times in the same person. Usual tears are slightly alkaline (and tend to become more so with corneal injuries) and average about pH 7.5 but may range from above pH 8 to below pH 6.

Bacteriostatic properties of tears

An enzyme, lysozyme, in tears, discovered by Fleming in 1922, possesses an antibacterial ability.[9] The enzyme is thought to act as a hydrolyzing agent on the wall of many bacteria. The lysozyme level in the tears is diminished by dilution from excessive tearing and in some associated pathologic conditions such as Sjögren's syndrome. The evaporation of tears when the eyes are open tends to lower the temperature of the cornea several degrees below the optimal temperature (35° to 38° C) for bacterial growth. This accounts in part for increased bacterial growth in eyes that are kept closed for extended periods.

Ford and co-workers[4] measured an antibacterial factor identical with or closely related to the β-lysin in human tears and human aqueous humor and found that its bactericidal activity was greater in human tears and in aqueous humor than in serum. They concluded that β-lysin is a normal constituent of human tears and aqueous humor and that it acts as an antibacterial agent in these fluids, possibly in concert with lysozyme in tears. The β-lysin appears to be similar or identical to an antibacterial nonlysozymal factor found in platelets, serum, and other body fluids.[7] Friedland and co-workers[5] isolated a nonlysozymal antibacterial factor from human tears that had a more powerful bactericidal activity than lysozyme. It was active against a wide spectrum of conjunctival inhabitants. They suggested that lysozyme does not kill bacteria in the tear film. The factor described probably is the β-lysin described by Ford and co-workers.[4]

TEAR FLOW

In the past much attention was focused on the proper drainage of tears from the eye, but now the importance of the tear film as it relates to the normal (and abnormal) function of the eye is being studied in much greater detail. The increasing use of contact lenses lends increased importance to these investigations.

The cornea and conjunctiva are kept moist by a continuous tear film. The tears are prevented from spilling over the cheek because of the oily secretion (chiefly from the meibomian glands) that is spread over the inner half of the lid margin. This secretion has a critical tension below that of the tears and hence is hydrophobic. Even the outer surface of the lid margin anterior to the orifices of the meibomian glands is hydrophobic, possibly because of the greasy, keratinized squamous cells.[10]

The corneal surface stays moist only when the mucin layer is in direct contact with the epithelium. The increased surface tension of the mucoid layer makes it hydrophilic, thus allowing the tear film to spread evenly over the cornea.

A meniscus of the lacrimal fluid collects at both the upper and lower lid margins of the cornea. The interaction of the lacrimal menisci and the adjacent thinner layer of lacrimal fluid can be observed with the use of the cobalt filter under high magnification after fluorescein is placed in the eye[11] (Fig. 2-1). As the eyelid closes, the thinned areas of the lacrimal film adjacent to the menisci of the upper and lower lids are pushed toward each other until they merge.

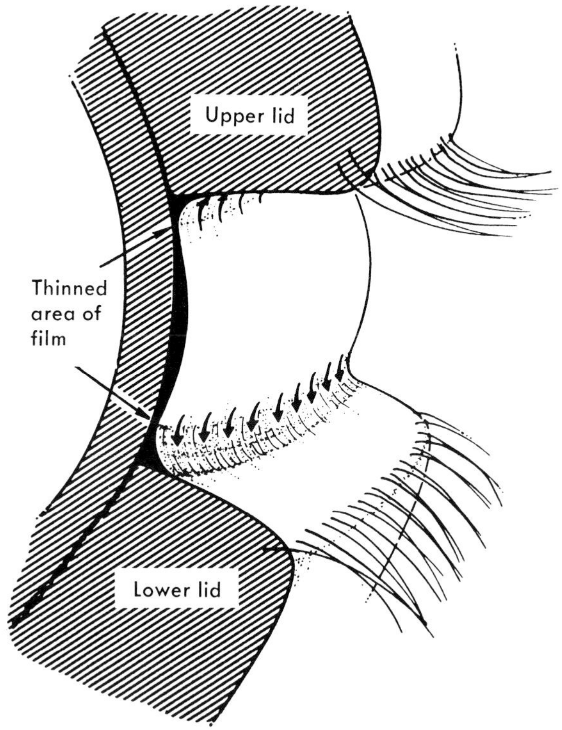

Fig. 2-1. Negative pressure in meniscus thins adjacent tear film. Blinking of eyelids acts as subsurface vacuum cleaner, resulting in renewal of aqueous phase of the tears. (From McDonald, J. E., and Brubaker, S.: Am J Ophthalmol **72**:139-146, 1971.)

With the opening of the eyelids, the tear film fractures in the area of meniscus-induced thinning, leaving a dry area of cornea that resists wetting. These dry areas may take the fluorescein stain. It is the negative pressure in the meniscus when the lids open that causes the thinning of the film. The fact that contact lenses are surrounded by a meniscus with an area of thinned film that may fracture (and leave a dry area on the cornea), may explain the staining frequently seen in the temporal and nasal portions of the exposed cornea.

The haziness that develops in corneas during prolonged exposure, as may occur during corneal transplantation or retinopexy, is probably due to corneal drying because the corneal epithelium is rendered hydrophobic after the removal of the mucin layer.

REMOVAL OF LACRIMAL SECRETIONS

The normal removal of tears is by evaporation and by drainage into the nose through the lacrimal drainage system. Because there are so many unknown and variable factors, estimation of the percentage of the tears that disappear through evaporation is highly speculative. If the average person secreted no more than

1 g or so of tears a day, as has been frequently quoted, a higher percentage of tears would be expected to be eliminated by evaporation than if 15 to 30 g were secreted, as has been suggested. The low secretor (such as an elderly person) who is exposed to a hot, dry atmosphere will have more evaporation of tears than will the profuse secretor in a cool, moist atmosphere.

Most of the tears enter the conjunctival sac under the upper lid; nearly all the tears secreted from the main lacrimal glands empty in the outer third of the eye, and most of the tears drain into the lower canaliculus.

Recent investigations[11] of the movement of tears suggest that gravity may play only a little role in the movement of tears. The sucking action of the eyelid menisci with blinking is the most plausible explanation for the vertical movement of tears. The tears are propelled in a nasal direction because with each closure of the lids the entire lid margin shifts nasally. The contraction of the tensor tarsus muscles may be the major factor in causing the nasal movement of the lid margin with eyelid closure. The tensor tarsus (Horner's) muscle (which has its origin along the posterior lacrimal crest, passes laterally forward, and after dividing into an upper and a lower slip, surrounds the canaliculi

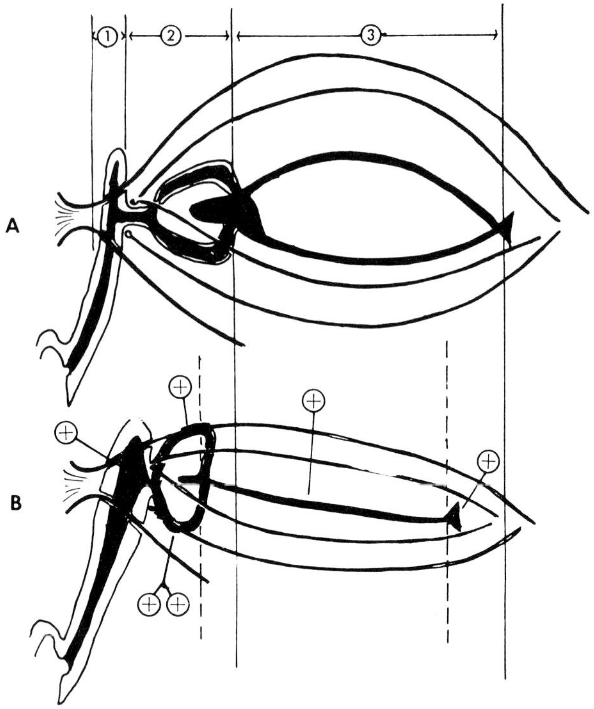

Fig. 2-2. Schematic representation of lacrimal pump. **A,** Eyelids open. **B,** Eyelids closed. *1,* Saccular pump; *2,* canalicular pump; *3,* palpebral pump. (From Worst, J. G. F.: Anatomic considerations in lacrimal sac surgery. In Veirs, E. R., editor: The lacrimal system: Proceedings of the first international symposium, St. Louis, 1971, The C. V. Mosby Co.)

to become continuous with the pretarsal portions of the orbicularis muscle having its origin from the medial palpebral ligament and surrounding bone) plays a part in the movement of the eyelid margin nasally with lid closure.

As shown schematically in Fig. 2-2, when the eyelids are open, a tear strip is present along the lid margin; the lacrimal canaliculi are distended and filled with fluid, and the lacrimal sac is only a potential space.[17] When the eyelids close, the upper and lower strips unite to form the retropalpebral canal, which has been shortened with the lid closure. This is termed the "palpebral pump," which exerts positive pressure on the eyelid in the retropalpebral canal and is present only during the short phase of eyelid closure. Contraction of muscles surrounding the lacrimal canaliculi causes the canaliculi to shorten and thereby exert positive pressure on their contents. The lower canaliculus is longer than the upper and shortens more than the upper. Contraction of the muscles on the outer wall of the lacrimal sac opens the sac and produces negative pressure. Worst[17] called the third phase of the lacrimal pump mechanism "the saccular pump." Tears within the lacrimal sac flow through the nasolacrimal duct into the nose with the opening of the eyelids that results in collapse of the sac.

The preceding description of the mechanism of tear drainage is plausible, but future investigations may uncover the precise factors responsible. Closure of the puncta during closure of the lid is probably an essential function in lid drainage. In a young child referred to me because of unilateral epiphora since birth the punctum on the side of the epiphora had a slitlike opening. The tissues of the punctum area, as well as the free margin extending medially from the punctum, were "paper thin." The lower punctum had a limited movement with opening and closing of the eyelids. The inability to close the punctum would seem the most likely cause of the epiphora; limited movement of the punctum may have played a part.

REFERENCES

1. Apt, L., and Cullen, B. F.: Newborns do secrete tears, JAMA 189:951-953, 1964.
2. Botelho, S. Y., Hisada, M., and Fuenmayor, N.: Functional innervation of the lacrimal gland in the cat, Arch Ophthalmol 76:581-588, 1966.
3. Duke-Elder, S.: Cited by Whitwell.[16]
4. Ford, L. C., DeLange, R. J., and Petty, R. W.: Identification of a nonlysozymal bactericidal factor (beta lysin) in human tears and aqueous humor, Am J Ophthalmol 81: 30-33, 1976.
5. Friedland, B. R., Anderson, D. R., and Forster, R. K.: Nonlysozyme antibacterial factor in human tears, Am J Ophthalmol 74:52-59, 1972.
6. Hashimoto, M., Otsuka, H., Chinen, Y., and Azuma, R.: A new Schirmer test using phenol-red paper strip, Folia Ophthalmol Jap 14:337-340, 1963.
7. Jensen, R. S., Tew, J. G., and Donaldson, D. M.: Extracellular β-lysin and muramidase in body fluids and inflammatory exudates, Proc Soc Exp Biol Med 124:545-549, 1967.
8. Jones, L. T., Reeh, M. J., and Wirtschafter, J. D.: Ophthalmic anatomy, Rochester, Minn., 1970, American Academy of Ophthalmology and Otolaryngology, p. 272.
9. Lewis, J. G., and Stephens, P. J.: Tear glucose in diabetics, Br J Ophthalmol 42:754-758, 1958.
10. McDonald, J. E.: Surface phenomena of tear films, Trans Am Ophthalmol Soc 66:905-939, 1968.

11. McDonald, J. E., and Brubaker, S.: Meniscus-induced thinning of tear films, Am J Ophthalmol 72:139-146, 1971.
12. Mastman, G. J., Baldes, E. J., and Henderson, J. W.: The total osmotic pressure of tears in normal and various pathologic conditions, Arch Ophthalmol 65:509-513, 1961.
13. Norm, M. S.: Tear secretion in normal eyes estimated by a new method: the lacrimal streak dilution test, Acta Ophthalmol 43:567-573, 1965.
14. Sapse, A. T., Bonavida, B., Stone, W., Jr., and Sercarz, E. E.: Human tear lysozyme. III. Preliminary study on lysozyme levels in subjects with smog eye irritation, Am J Ophthalmol 66:76-80, 1968.
15. Stiewe, M.: The age factor in lacrimation, Z Alternsforsch 15:318-323, 1962.
16. Whitwell, J.: Role of the sympathetic in lacrimal secretion, Br J Ophthalmol 45:439-445, 1961.
17. Worst, J. G. F.: Anatomic considerations in lacrimal sac surgery. In Veirs, E. R., editor: The lacrimal system, proceedings of the first international symposium, St. Louis, 1971, The C. V. Mosby Co., pp. 98-117.

CHAPTER 3

Secretory disorders of the lacrimal system

The eye is kept comfortable and capable of performing its function when there is continuous moistening of the cornea and conjunctiva with the proper quantity and quality of tears. The tears have additional functions such as washing foreign material from the conjunctival sac and cornea and providing protection against infection. The tear film consists of (1) the inner or mucin layer (the layer that is essential to the optics of the eye and that provides a base for the tears), (2) the middle or tear layer, and (3) the oily layer, which functions to prevent tears from spilling over the eyelid margin and diminishes the rate of evaporation of tears from the eye.

Tears are secreted by the main and accessory lacrimal glands; these glands have an efferent parasympathetic nerve supply. The main lacrimal gland is the large gland. The conjunctival and tarsal glands and the accessory glands of Krause and of Wolfring plus the oil gland do not have an efferent nerve supply; these glands have been called the basic secretors.

It has been postulated that the basic secretors supply the normal tear fluid and that the main lacrimal gland with its efferent nerve supply functions essentially as a reflex response—that is, it secretes only when there is eye irritation such as with foreign bodies on the cornea or an emotional experience. There is little evidence to support this theory.

FUNCTIONAL EXAMINATION OF LACRIMAL SYSTEM

Functional testing of the lacrimal system, properly performed in the proper sequence, is essential in the correct evaluation of disorders of the lacrimal drainage system. There are many pathologic conditions that cause symptoms, and sometimes there are multiple disorders in the same patient. Time, patience, and awareness of the abnormal conditions that can be responsible for symptoms are necessary. Without proper and thorough examination, the patient may be subjected to treatment that has no chance of relieving the symptoms. For example, if fluid enters the nose during irrigation, one might conclude that spontaneous drainage of tears should occur. However, fluid may enter the nose during irrigation in patients who have partial stenosis of the common canaliculus or who have dacryoliths. The dye test or a dacryocystogram, as well as other tests, could be most helpful in arriving at the proper diagnosis.

Dye test

The instillation of drops of 0.5% to 2% fluorescein into the conjunctival sac or the use of moistened fluorescein strips (generally used in checking applanation intraocular pressure) is the most useful but most neglected method of determining whether tears flow spontaneously from the conjunctival sac into the nose. After instillation of the fluorescein into the conjunctival sac, the patient's head is bent forward. A nasal metal applicator with a small wisp of moistened cotton on its tip is passed beneath the anterior tip of the lower nasal turbinate. Some facility in the use of a head mirror is essential. If no dye shows on the cotton-tipped applicator, the patient is asked to hold one nostril closed and blow into a white paper napkin; then the maneuver is repeated with the other nostril closed. If dye is blown out of a nostril, that is proof that tears drain spontaneously on that side. Gentle lavage of the lower level of the nose with isotonic saline to obtain evidence of dye entering the nose spontaneously also can be tried.

In most young persons with normally functioning drainage systems the fluorescein will stain the cotton on the applicator within 1 to 2 minutes. With less efficient drainage systems or with decreased tear formation, several minutes may be required before the dye is detected in the nose. Tear drainage into the nose apparently does occur in a few symptomless persons who have no demonstrable dye flow.

The dye test can be used to determine if the position of the lower punctum is such that tears are capable of entering the canaliculus. With the patient's head held upright, a small amount of fluorescein is instilled in the temporal aspect of the cul-de-sac. If the lower punctum is turned outward, often to a minimal degree, it can be easily seen that the fluorescein does not reach to it. Neither can the tears in these cases. This test should be performed prior to instillation of fluorescein to determine if fluorescein enters the nose. If fluorescein is instilled into the conjunctival cul-de-sac on both sides simultaneously, frequently the dye can be seen to spill over the cheek on the side that has no spontaneous drainage of tears into the nose.

Ocular staining tests

Rose bengal is used almost exclusively for this test (the staining pattern will be altered if the test is done after the Schirmer test or after instillation of topical anesthetic). One drop of 1% rose bengal is instilled into each conjunctival sac, followed by irrigation with isotonic saline; the patients may complain of a moderate burning sensation that soon disappears. When keratoconjunctivitis sicca is significantly severe, the exposed portion of the bulbar conjunctiva stains a brilliant red, more marked in the lower part of the palpebral aperture. The conjunctiva of the palpebral aperture stains in two triangular areas, nasal and temporal, with their bases at the limbus. The cornea, especially the lower two thirds, shows stained corneal cells. Threads of mucus may be seen adhering to the cornea. Many normal eyes will stain lightly.

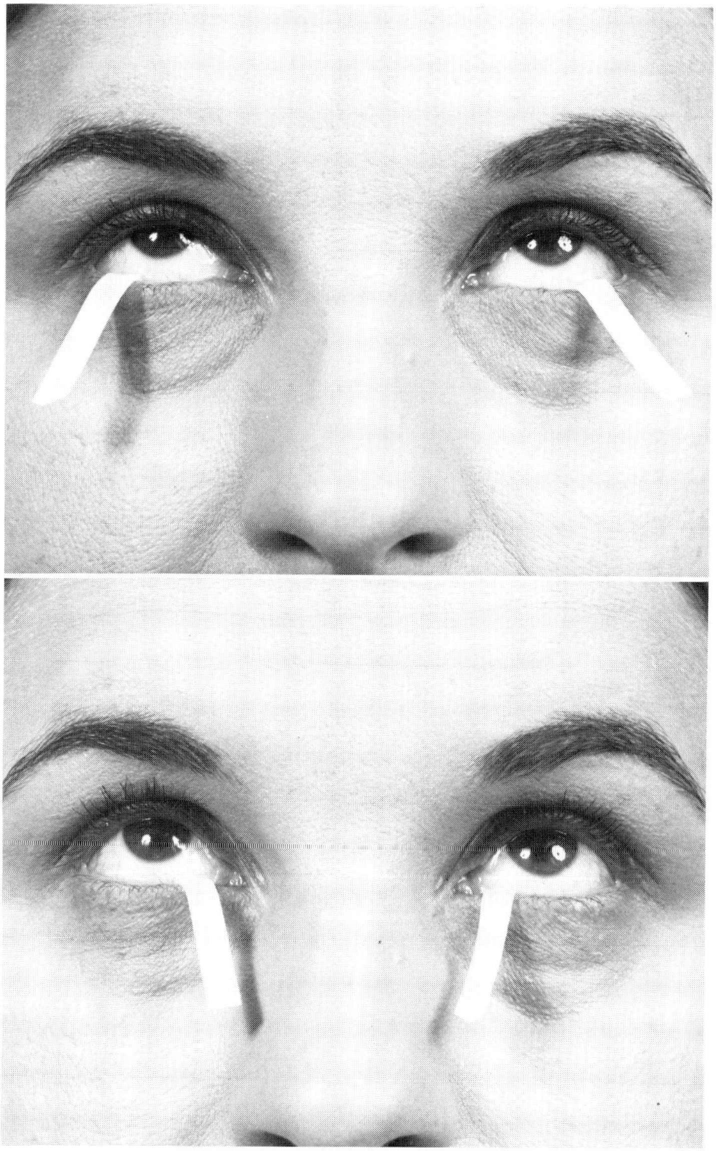

Fig. 3-1. Schirmer test. *Top,* Filter paper inserted laterally. Patient is asked to look upward. *Bottom,* Filter paper inserted on nasal side.

The Schirmer test

This test is easily, quickly, and inexpensively performed. Although not highly accurate, it does provide much valuable information. Whatman no. 41 filter paper is cut into strips 5 mm wide and about 35 mm long. One end is folded so that about 5 mm can be tucked within the lower lid, near either the inner or outer canthus (Fig. 3-1). The measurement of the amount of wetting includes only the exposed portion of the filter paper. The average amount of wetting for a normal young person is usually given as about 15 mm in 5 minutes. Many symptomless patients, especially elderly ones, may show no more than 5 mm of wetting in 5 minutes. Although Sjögren's syndrome cannot be diagnosed by the Schirmer test alone, evidence of dry eyes alerts the examiner that further tests for this disease may be in order.

In a modification of the Schirmer test the eye is anesthetized with a topical anesthetic. The amount of wetting is then measured by irritating the nasal mucosa. This test is used when the unmodified Schirmer test shows little wetting. It should measure the amount of reflex secretion produced by the main lacrimal glands.

Unless there is some contraindication, both sides should be tested simultaneously. If there is unilateral interference to proper tear drainage, the Schirmer test usually will show significantly more wetting on the side of the interference. This may be an important diagnostic clue. Patients who show 20 to 30 mm of wetting bilaterally in a period of a minute or less are obviously overproducing tears. This should alert the ophthalmologist that procedures designed to improve tear drainage may show disappointing results. This is especially true if fluorescein flows spontaneously into the nose.

Lavage

Many ophthalmologists who examine the lacrimal drainage system for patency will first lavage and if fluid is forced into the nose will conclude that tears should drain satisfactorily. Lavaging fluid into the nose proves only that fluid can be *forced* through the drainage passages. Many of these patients will have no spontaneous drainage of tears.

The punctum, usually the lower, is gently dilated with a punctum dilator only enough to allow the lacrimal tip to enter. Isotonic saline is instilled from the 2-ml syringe to which the lacrimal tip is attached. The upper lid is held up with one hand (or by an assistant) while the fluid is irrigated into the lower canaliculus. The patient holds an emesis basin under his nose with his head held forward so that the contents of the sac (if any) may be lavaged into the basin. Occasionally, a plug of mucus that has been obstructing drainage through the nasolacrimal duct will be lavaged into the basin. Rarely, obstruction caused by a fungal infection will be lavaged loose.

If some saline can be lavaged into the nose but simultaneously much of it exits through the upper canaliculus, partial obstruction of the common canalic-

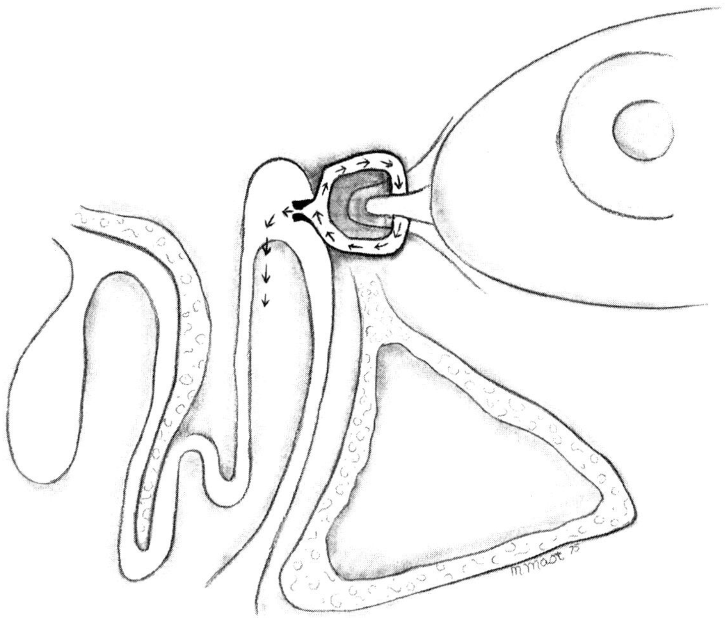

Fig. 3-2. Diagram explaining why epiphora occurs with partially stenosed common canaliculus. Because of partial stenosis, tears will not enter the sac spontaneously. Fluid injected into lower canaliculus under mild pressure will enter the tear sac (and nose) in part; remainder will exit through upper canaliculus. Eversion of upper punctum permits observation of fluid exiting there as fluid is injected into lower punctum.

ulus is usually present. If most of the fluid exits from the upper punctum, this is an exceedingly important observation (Fig. 3-2). These patients usually will have little or no spontaneous drainage of fluid into the nose, as shown by the dye test. Epiphora often is quite annoying unless the amount of tears secreted by the patient is decreased. This condition tends to develop in persons who are middle-age or older because the lumen of the canaliculus may develop a progressive narrowing, especially near the lacrimal sac.

If all the saline lavaged into the lower canaliculus immediately exits through the upper canaliculus, the obstruction is likely to be in the ampullary portion of the common canaliculus (Fig. 3-3).

When a patient has a small lacrimal sac obstructed inferiorly, all the saline seems to exit from the upper canaliculus immediately after it is lavaged through the lower. This erroneously suggests obstruction in the ampullary portion of the common canaliculus. Often, a small amount of mucoid material (easily overlooked) also will exit through the upper canaliculus in these cases. Furthermore, the patient is more likely to have a history suggestive of infection when there is a small obstructed sac. Dacryocystography should be performed in instances of doubt.

A

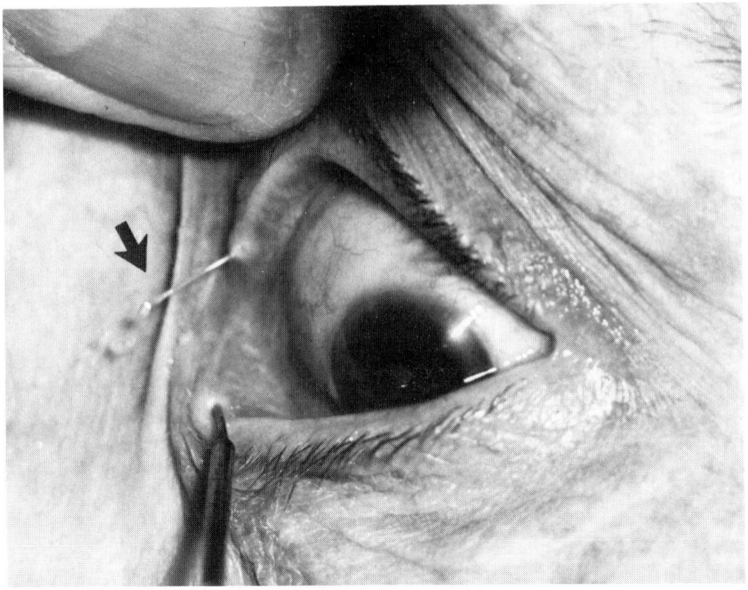

B

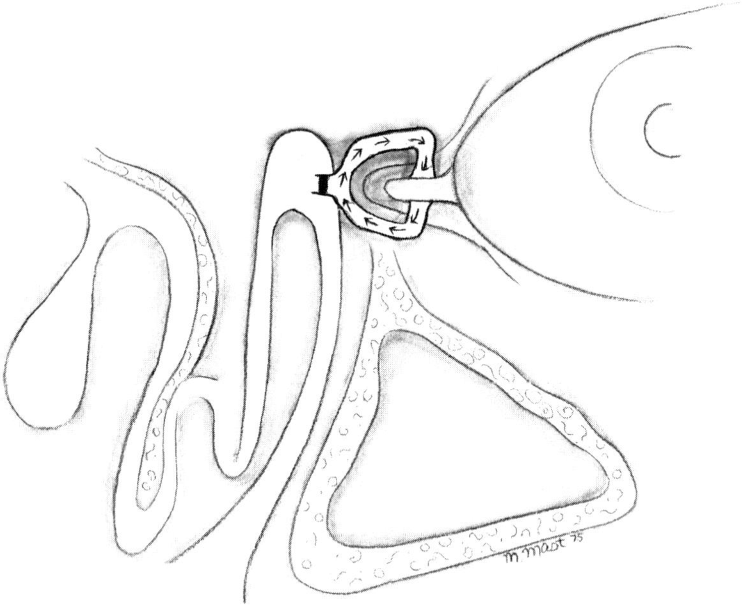

Fig. 3-3. Total obstruction of ampullary portion of canaliculus. **A,** Tinted fluid injected into lower canaliculus exits entirely from upper punctum *(arrow);* none enters nose. **B,** Path of injected fluid.

If fluid exits only through the canaliculus being lavaged, the obstruction is distal to the common canaliculus or involves all of the common canaliculus.

Taste test

The taste test to determine the drainage of tears is a subjective test that has not been widely used. Lipsius[4] recommended the use of 10% saccharin solution as a taste test. Hornblass[3] recommended instilling 1% saccharin solution into the conjunctival cul-de-sac and testing each eye at intervals of not less than 30 minutes. A drop of topical anesthetic is instilled prior to instilling the saccharin solution. Hornblass believes that the test is particularly useful for children as soon as they are old enough to give a valid response.

Test for tonicity of eyelid muscles

Diminished action of the lid muscles is easily determined. The orbicularis oculi muscles are the principal muscles responsible for adequate tear drainage. If the muscles are functioning properly, the inferior punctum will move nasally about 3 or 4 mm when the lids are in the act of closing. The lower punctum is difficult to observe during closure of the eyelids, even if the lid muscles are weak. A simple method to determine how much, if any, the lower punctum moves medially is to hold both eyelids upward and ask the patient to try to force his eyes closed. The movement of the puncta nasally can be easily determined. Also, the actual strength of the muscles can be estimated.

Probing

Probing has limited diagnostic value in studying the lacrimal drainage system. Often, lacrimal probes are used simultaneously as a therapeutic measure (for obstruction at the ampullary portion of the common canaliculus or for congenital obstruction of the nasolacrimal duct in infants). Probing for the purpose of dilating a stenosed canaliculus or nasolacrimal duct in adults is seldom of therapeutic value and often is harmful.

Usually a no. 0 or 00 Bowman probe is most satisfactory—seldom should a probe larger than no. 1 be used. Utmost gentleness should be exercised in passing the probe because unnecessary trauma may aggravate the problem. Dipping the tip of the probe in an ointment (ophthalmic ointments are nearly always readily available) may minimize the trauma.

Usually, the punctum must be dilated with a punctum dilator before a probe will enter the canaliculus. If the punctum is extremely small, a sharp-pointed dilator or safety pin may be needed. In passing a probe, it should be kept in mind that the canaliculus first runs vertically and then horizontally. The total length of the canaliculi is in the range of 8.5 to 10 mm, the upper being slightly shorter than the lower. After the probe is passed through the vertical portion of the canaliculus, the lid should be stretched laterally until the probe hits an obstruction—the medial wall of the lacrimal sac if there is no obstruction. If the nasolacrimal duct is to be probed, the probe should be held snugly against the nasal bone with the eyelid pulled laterally. The lateral pull on the lid is gradually released as the probe is carefully brought into a nearly vertical direction and passed through the nasolacrimal duct.

LACRIMAL HYPERSECRETION

Hypersecretion of tears is secretion of more than the normal amount of tears; epiphora is the condition in which tears overflow the eyelids and may be due to faulty drainage. Apparent hypersecretion of tears may be the result of blockage of the tear drainage system. If epiphora is unilateral, the odds are strongly in favor of blockage on the offending side rather than hypersecretion. The fluorescein dye test is most helpful: if the fluorescein instilled into the conjunctival sac flows into the nose spontaneously, hypersecretion is the cause of the patient's tearing. Quantitative studies[5] have shown that the main lacrimal gland has 50 times more acini than are found in all the accessory lacrimal glands combined (Fig. 3-4). The excess secretion of tears comes from that gland.

Excess tear formation can be extremely annoying to some, such as the highly nervous person and the person who experiences much exposure to cold, windy weather. The tears well up in the conjunctival sac, blurring vision; they re-form soon after the eyes are wiped. The lower lid margins may become irritated, and the adjacent skin may become macerated. However, in contrast to excessively dry eyes, the excessive wetness offers no threat to the integrity of the eye.

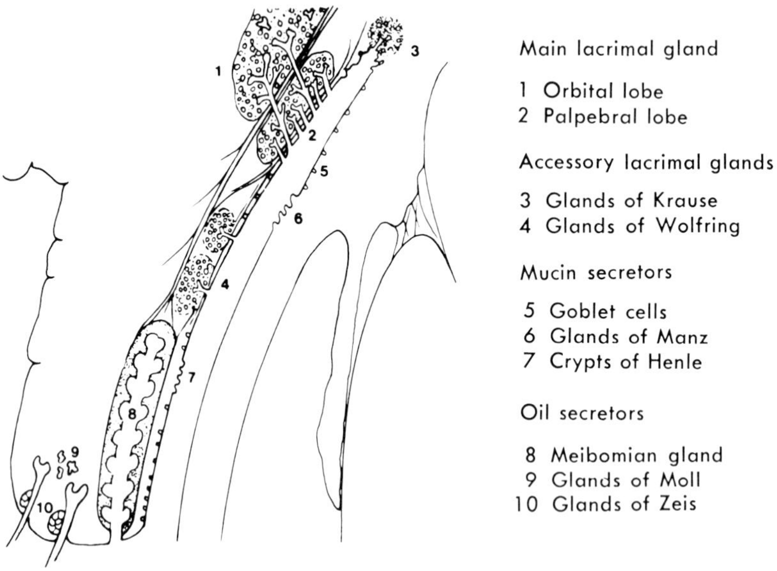

Fig. 3-4. Schematic representation of secretory tear system. (From Scherz, W., and Dohlman, C. H.: Arch Ophthalmol 93:281-283, 1975.)

Etiology. Hypersecretion of the lacrimal gland can be due to various causes. At times the hypersecretion is a symptom of a serious general disorder. The patient may consult the ophthalmologist first.

Disorders of the thyroid gland, including both hyperthyroidism and hypothyroidism, are frequently associated with excess tear secretion. With toxic thyroid disease that has its onset in older persons (past 50 or 60 years of age), the onset often is not dramatic, and the signs and symptoms are subtle. These patients frequently will complain of increased nervousness and loss of weight. The Schirmer test frequently shows a marked increase in tear formation. If no adequate explanation can be found for the excess tearing in such patients, they should be referred to an internist or at the minimum undergo some basic thyroid function tests.

Nervous persons are prone to oversecrete—often intermittently. A difficult type of hypersecretion to treat is that which occurs in older persons with marked arteriosclerosis. These are the weepy patients who have frequent emotional outbursts without any rational cause.

Local disorders of the eye, and especially of the cornea, such as ulcers, foreign bodies, intraocular disease, and numerous other local irritative lesions are common causes of excessive reflex hypersecretion. Disorders of the adjacent structures, sinuses, nose (common cold) and allergies, for example, and to a lesser degree other lesions in the area, may stimulate excessive tear formation.

Lacrimation, at times profuse, may occur with lesions involving the lacrimal gland, such as tumors and inflammatory processes. Even if not adjacent to the gland, inflammatory lesions of the orbit may cause hypersecretion of tears.

Treatment. The ideal treatment is directed at the cause, if possible. If this approach is ineffective, the decision is made whether to advise the patient to accept the annoyance of excessive tearing or to resort to a procedure to decrease the rate of secretion. Several factors should be considered.

If the symptoms are reasonably acceptable to the patient, he should live with the annoyance. Operative measures to permanently decrease the amount of tear secretion are more logically performed in the older age group, especially if symptoms have been present for a considerable time. Hypersecretion often will spontaneously diminish without apparent reason, and if this were to happen in a younger patient who had already undergone an operation to decrease tear secretion, keratoconjunctivitis sicca could be the unpleasant permanent sequela. Also, normally there is a slow diminution of tear secretion with aging, another reason for a conservative approach in the young. The younger patient would have a longer time to develop an excessively dry eye and a longer period to suffer the same. Scherz and Dohlman[5] reported persistent keratoconjunctivitis sicca developing immediately after a palpebral dacryoadenectomy in a healthy 43-year-old woman with normal eyes and tear function prior to the operation. Ten years after the operation the affected eye continued to show the classic

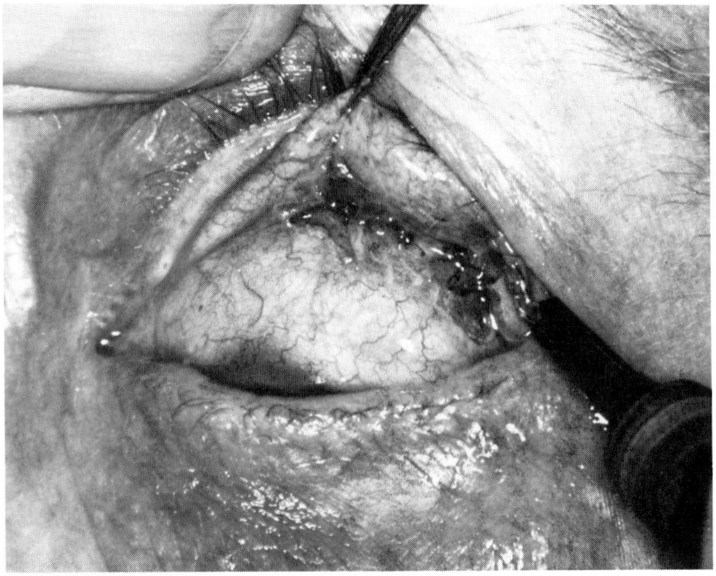

Fig. 3-5. Cauterization of ductules to decrease secretion. Cautery is applied to upper 3 mm of superior temporal (outer) half of bulbar conjunctiva to permanently seal some of ductules from lacrimal gland. Procedure can be repeated.

signs and symptoms of a keratoconjunctivitis sicca. The authors mentioned several other reports of similar situations.

In 33 cases analyzed by Taiara and Smith[8] (follow-up: range, 2 months to 5¾ years; mean, 12 months), palpebral dacryoadenectomy was considered successful in 19 cases and unsuccessful in 14. A mild xerophthalmia was reported in one patient; the Schirmer test result was 0, but no symptoms were apparent 3 years later. A follow-up period of 5 years as a minimum, and preferably 10 or more years, might dampen one's enthusiasm for this procedure.

In my experience, removing the palpebral lobe of the lacrimal gland has not been consistently successful. Another procedure is available to decrease tear formation and has the advantage that the amount can be graduated. This involves using a small ball-point cautery tip to close off the ductules from the lacrimal gland (Fig. 3-5). These ductules from the main and palpebral lobes empty into the conjunctival sac just anteriorly to the lateral half of the upper cul-de-sac. At best, cautery will not close off all the ductules because one or more open near the outer canthus or a little below the outer canthus. This procedure can be repeated after a few months if the tear secretion is not sufficiently decreased.

Comment. Hypersecretion of lacrimal tears is a fairly common complaint among ophthalmologic patients. Accurate determination of the cause and treatment of the cause, if one can be found and is treatable, is the most logical approach. The best advice to give any patient, and especially the younger ones, is to live with the annoyance because the amount of tears secreted usually diminishes with age, although this improvement may not occur before middle age or later. Those with excessive tearing due to thyroid disorders often notice improvement as their thyroid problem resolves.

Operative measures, especially removal of the palpebral lobe of the lacrimal gland, may be used in the more severe cases in elderly patients (past age 65 years). Fewer than half these patients will get a reasonable amount of relief. An occasional case of keratoconjunctivitis sicca will develop, and they will wish they had their tears back. Cautery of the upper cul-de-sac is less likely to result in keratoconjunctivitis sicca than is removal of the palpebral lobe of the gland.

LACRIMAL HYPOSECRETION

The newborn infant starts life with minimal tear secretion, but the rate of secretion develops rapidly. After middle age, the rate progressively diminishes as a normal physiologic process. Many elderly persons in their eighth or ninth decade or older may have 2 to 3 mm of moistening as measured with the Schirmer test and yet have minimal or no symptoms of dryness. Conversely, many highstrung young persons will have a chief complaint of dry eyes but 20 mm or more of moistening on the Schirmer test. There may be two primary tear deficiencies: (1) such as occurs in keratoconjunctivitis sicca in rheumatoid arthritis and (2) a mucus deficiency in conditions such as Stevens-Johnson syndrome, early pemphigoid, and avitaminosis A.

A marked decrease in tear formation may occur if only the palpebral lobe of the lacrimal gland is removed or if the palpebral and orbital lobes are extirpated. About 50% of patients will experience some decrease of tear secretion immediately after removal of the palpebral lobe alone. After this procedure a sufficient number of patients will have no tears measurable by the Schirmer test to cause one to think twice about using this procedure, except for marked hypersecretion not responsive to other measures—and only in older patients.

Sjögren's syndrome

In 1933 Hendrik Sjögren described a condition and suggested the disease he described be called "keratoconjunctivitis sicca" (dry eyes). The term "Sjögren's syndrome" is probably applicable when keratoconjunctivitis sicca is associated with (1) recurrent or chronic "idiopathic" salivary gland swelling, (2) unexplained xerostomia, and (3) connective tissue disease, especially rheumatoid arthritis. Shearn[6] stated that in many patients with Sjögren's syndrome arthritis never develops, even though these patients may also have such "immunologic" diseases as thyroiditis, biliary cirrhosis, or purpura hyperglobulinemia. About 14% of rheumatoid patients have keratoconjunctivitis sicca as diagnosed by the rose bengal test; about 25% of patients with keratoconjunctivitis sicca have rheumatoid arthritis.

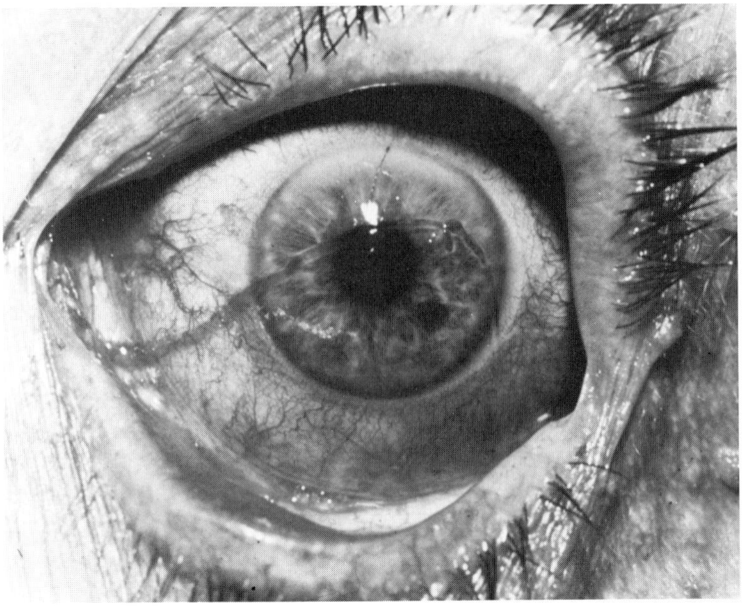

Fig. 3-6. Keratoconjunctivitis sicca with filaments. Intense red staining is seen only as darkened conjunctiva in palpebral aperture. No measurable tears with Schirmer test. Patient had Sjögren's syndrome.

Sjögren's syndrome has a marked predilection for women; the male-to-female ratio is about 1:9. The onset is in middle age or later. All patients I have seen complained significantly about their dry eyes; additional complaints included photophobia, a scratchy, burning sensation, and sticky secretion. Many of the patients are said to have few eye symptoms with the dry eyes and staining corneas. When the proper diagnosis is not made, irritative eye drops often are prescribed, which only aggravates the symptoms.

Diagnosis. Along with dry eyes, patients with Sjögren's syndrome have dry membranes elsewhere (nose, mouth, and throat). The eye signs and symptoms are almost always bilateral. These eyes are best examined under a slitlamp, which permits one to see the markedly diminished tear strip at the lower lid margin and small clumps of debris on the cornea. If filaments are present, they seem to be adhering to the cornea. These filaments are produced by the goblet cell of the conjunctiva. When 1% rose bengal is instilled into the eye (warn the patient that the solution will burn) followed by lavage with isotonic saline, fairly marked staining will occur on the lower two thirds of the cornea with lesser amounts of staining of the bulbar conjunctiva of the interpalpebral tissue (Fig. 3-6).

Pathology. The major lacrimal glands are massively infiltrated with lymphocytes and plasma cells, causing extreme atrophy of the secretory acini. The secretory ability of the accessory lacrimal glands is likewise destroyed. Fortunately, the goblet cells furnish the mucin layer, the oil gland still functions, and probably some aqueous permeates the cornea to be of some aid. The bulbar conjunctiva is involved in the deterioration. Filamentary keratitis occurs as the disease progresses. Corneal perforation can occur.

In an excellent study to correlate ocular findings and labial salivary gland histology, Tabbara and co-workers[7] found that of the patients with grade 4 lymphocytic infiltration of their labial salivary tissues more than 90% had decreased or no tear lysozyme content. There was also a high correlation between the severity of the keratoconjunctivitis sicca in patients with Sjögren's syndrome and the degree of infiltration of the labial salivary tissues. An interesting finding was that all of the 26 patients were women. In contrast, 73% of the patients with rheumatoid arthritis were men.

Allen and co-workers[1] have shown that in the human gland the type A cell (K or mucous cell) makes up more of the gland volume than does the type B cell (G or serous cell).

Treatment. Treatment is symptomatic and usually very discouraging. Cure is never achieved; remission is rare. The various artificial tear solutions give a little relief. Irrigating the eyes with balanced salt solution affords some patients temporary respite. Closing the puncta to retain the patient's tears is disappointing because these patients usually do not secrete any tears. Theoretically, closing the puncta would help retain the artificial tears instilled into the conjunctival sac for a longer period.

Closing the puncta, usually by cautery, is not recommended except in patients who have permanently dry eyes as in Sjögren's syndrome or in young patients in whom the dryness is due to removal of the lacrimal gland. Patients are seen who complain of dry eyes and show little tear formation by the Schirmer test, and for whose condition there is no adequate explanation. Later, many of these patients become symptomless and will exhibit adequate tear formation.

Miscellaneous causes of hyposecretion

These include benign mucosal pemphigoid, also known as essential shrinkage of the conjunctiva. It is a rare, chronic, progressive disease that involves the conjunctiva as well as the oral mucosa. The scarring results in closure of the ductules from the main lacrimal gland as well as the accessory lacrimal gland. The mucin deficiency occurs as goblet cells are destroyed. Accompanying the dry eyes is trichiasis and neovascularization and ulceration of the cornea.

The progressive loss of vision (to blindness at times) and the constant discomfort of the eyes is a distressing chain of events. No cause is known, and treatment is purely symptomatic. Patients will at times put a drop of water into their eyes every few minutes; a balanced salt solution might be preferable. Soft contact lens may provide more comfort.

In sarcoidosis, inflammation of the lacrimal gland destroys the acini that secrete the tears. Evidence of sarcoidosis in other parts of the body or biopsy of the lacrimal gland confirms the diagnosis; there is no ideal treatment. Use of artificial tears, as for dry eyes from other conditions, may give symptomatic relief.

Cook and co-workers[2] treated two patients by using alternate-day prednisone therapy. One patient had increased tear formation, which relieved the eye irritation from dryness; the second patient's markedly enlarged lacrimal glands returned to normal size.

Trachoma is a common cause for hyposecretion of tears where the disease is widespread.

Numerous neurogenic lesions, such as supranuclear facial nerve lesions, may result in decreased tear formation.

The secretory elements of the lacrimal gland may be severely affected by atrophic or cicatricial changes occurring with general disease and age.

Children with familial dysautonomia (Riley-Day syndrome) have many other congenital anomalies in addition to their alacrima, including blotching of the skin, arterial hypertension, marked emotional instability, and muscular hypotonia.

Rarely, hyposecretion of tears or alacrima occurs as an isolated congenital anomaly.

REFERENCES

1. Allen, M., Wright, P., and Reid, L.: The human lacrimal gland. A histochemical and organ culture study of the secretory cells, Arch Ophthalmol 88:493-497, 1972.
2. Cook, J. R., Brubaker, R. F., Jonathan, S., and Sheagren, J.: Lacrimal sarcoidosis treated with corticosteroids, Arch Ophthalmol 88:513-517, 1972.
3. Hornblass, A.: A simple taste test for lacrimal obstruction, Arch Ophthalmol 90:435-436, 1973.
4. Lipsius, E. I.: Sodium saccharin for testing the patency of the lacrimal passages, Am J Ophthalmol 41:320, 1956.
5. Scherz, W., and Dohlman, C. H.: Is the lacrimal gland dispensable? Keratoconjunctivitis sicca after lacrimal gland removal, Arch Ophthalmol 93:281-283, 1975.
6. Shearn, M. A.: Sjögren's syndrome, Philadelphia, 1971, W. B. Saunders Company.
7. Tabbara, K. F., Ostler, H. B., Daniels, T. E., Sylvester, R. A., Greenspan, J. S., and Talai, N.: Sjögren's syndrome: A correlation between ocular findings and labial salivary gland histology, Trans Am Acad Ophthalmol Otolaryngol 78:467-478, 1974.
8. Taiara, C., and Smith, B.: Palpebral dacryoadenectomy, Am J Ophthalmol 75:461-465, 1973.

CHAPTER 4

Congenital abnormalities

Congenital anomalies are understandably common along the course of the lacrimal drainage system and rare in the secretory parts of the system. During development, when the maxillary process overlaps the nasal process, a column of epithelial cells is buried along this line. The canaliculi will originate as an outbudding at the upper end of this column. Late in the embryonic stage there is a canalization of this solid column of cells to form the puncta, the canaliculi, the lacrimal sac, and the nasolacrimal duct emptying into the nose below the inferior turbinate.

A large number of congenital anomalies may occur along this drainage channel, the most common being congenital occlusion of the nasolacrimal duct. This may be because normally the thin membrane at the nasal extremity of this duct does not disappear until shortly before or after birth.

Except for congenital occlusions of the nasolacrimal duct, congenital anomalies of the lacrimal system are relatively uncommon. Many are asymptomatic. The symptomatic anomalies may be simple to correct or quite complicated.

Heredity plays a role in a few instances. In one family all three siblings had congenital absence of all the canaliculi, and one of the three also had congenital occlusion of the nasolacrimal duct, which caused enormously enlarged sacs. Another patient had a unilateral noninflammatory enlargement of the lacrimal sac with congenital occlusion of the canaliculus and closure of the nasolacrimal duct.

Patients with congenital anomalies of the lacrimal system may have congenital anomalies of other parts of the body, for example, anhidrotic ectodermal dysplasia.[1] Turner[6] reported five patients with congenital lacrimal duct obstruction among 22 patients with congenital glaucoma.

OCCLUSION OF NASOLACRIMAL DUCT

Frequency. The thin membrane that occludes the nasal end of the nasolacrimal duct during embryonic life disappears in the majority of infants by the time of birth. Of the approximately one third of infants in whom this membrane has not disappeared at birth, only in 2% to 4% will it persist sufficiently long to be clinically evident—that is, about 7 days. Heredity may be a factor in some instances. Persistent occlusions are probably more common in the first- and second-born siblings.

Signs. Because the secretion of tears may be minimal in the newborn infant, the characteristic signs of pooling of tears at the inner canthal region and epiphora may not be noticed until the infant is 1 or more weeks of age. Infection resulting from stagnation of tears may require several days to be discerned clinically.

The infection that develops with persistent occlusion of the duct can vary in degree. Minimally, the conjunctiva is mildly injected, and a small amount of mucoid secretion is present that frequently causes the lids to be "matted" together after sleep. In more severe infections these signs are more pronounced. In some cases digital pressure over the lacrimal sac causes regurgitation of mucopus from the lacrimal sac into the conjunctival sac. Signs of congenital occlusion of the nasolacrimal duct are easier to recognize if the condition is unilateral.

Acute dacryocystitis, as evidenced by swelling of the lacrimal sac, develops only rarely in the very young. When the lacrimal sac is swollen at birth, accumulation of epithelial, mucoid, and other material, rather than infection, is the

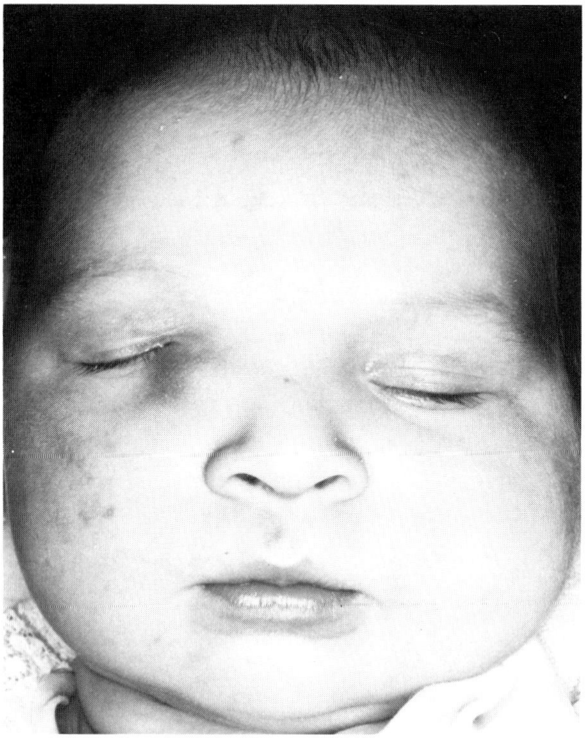

Fig. 4-1. Appearance of benign tumor, present since birth, resembles that of acute dacryocystitis secondary to congenital occlusion of nasolacrimal duct.

likely cause, although infection is superimposed early unless nasolacrimal patency is established.

Benign tumors may closely resemble acute dacryocystitis (Fig. 4-1). Some tumors will have a bluish appearance (hemangioma); with others, the appearance of the overlying skin is normal. Clinically, the absence of epiphora or mucopus and the inability to reduce the tumor by massage make involvement of the lacrimal sac highly unlikely. All such benign tumors that I have followed have disappeared spontaneously after a few months.

Treatment. Some flexible guidelines may be useful not only to ophthalmologists but also to pediatricians and others who see these patients.

If all conservative measures fail in the very young, an external dacryocystorhinostomy should be performed at an older age, preferably after age 3 to 3½ years.

Conservative treatment is usually indicated during the first 3 months or so of life. Spontaneous cures are frequent during this period, whereas after this age the percentage of spontaneous cure diminishes rapidly. Another reason for waiting until the infant is 3 months of age is that the puncta, canaliculi, and associated structures are larger, making probing easier. Mild antiseptic drops, such as sodium sulfacetamide, or antibiotic drops instilled into the conjunctival sac several times a day may help keep conjunctival infection under better control. If secretions or purulent material accumulates within the lacrimal sac, application of digital pressure over the sac two or three times a day may keep the eye from getting too "messy."

Probing. Probing is indicated in infants whose nasolacrimal duct has not opened spontaneously during the first 3 or 4 months of life. Probing may be advisable before this time if (1) the infection is considerable, especially if there is evidence of swelling of the lacrimal sac, (2) the parents are unduly apprehensive, or (3) it seems likely the infant might not be brought in as directed for further observation. In doubtful situations, such as those with minimal signs suggestive of obstruction, irrigation with isotonic saline to determine patency is indicated. If obstruction is confirmed, probing can then be done.

Probing of congenitally obstructed nasolacrimal ducts may be successful up to 12 to 18 months of age and occasionally at an older age. At these later ages there often are cicatricial changes that result in much lower percentages of success.

Tragically, many infants with congenital occlusion of the nasolacrimal duct are not treated by proper probing or at a sufficiently early age when success of probing should be nearly 100%. Often, this is due to the parents' failure to seek medical attention, but not infrequently physicians not familiar with the importance of early attention postpone early referral to an ophthalmologist.

Complications. Failure to effect permanent patency of the nasolacrimal duct is the most common problem. This failure is due to improper technique in probing in the vast majority of instances. In rare cases failure may occur in infants

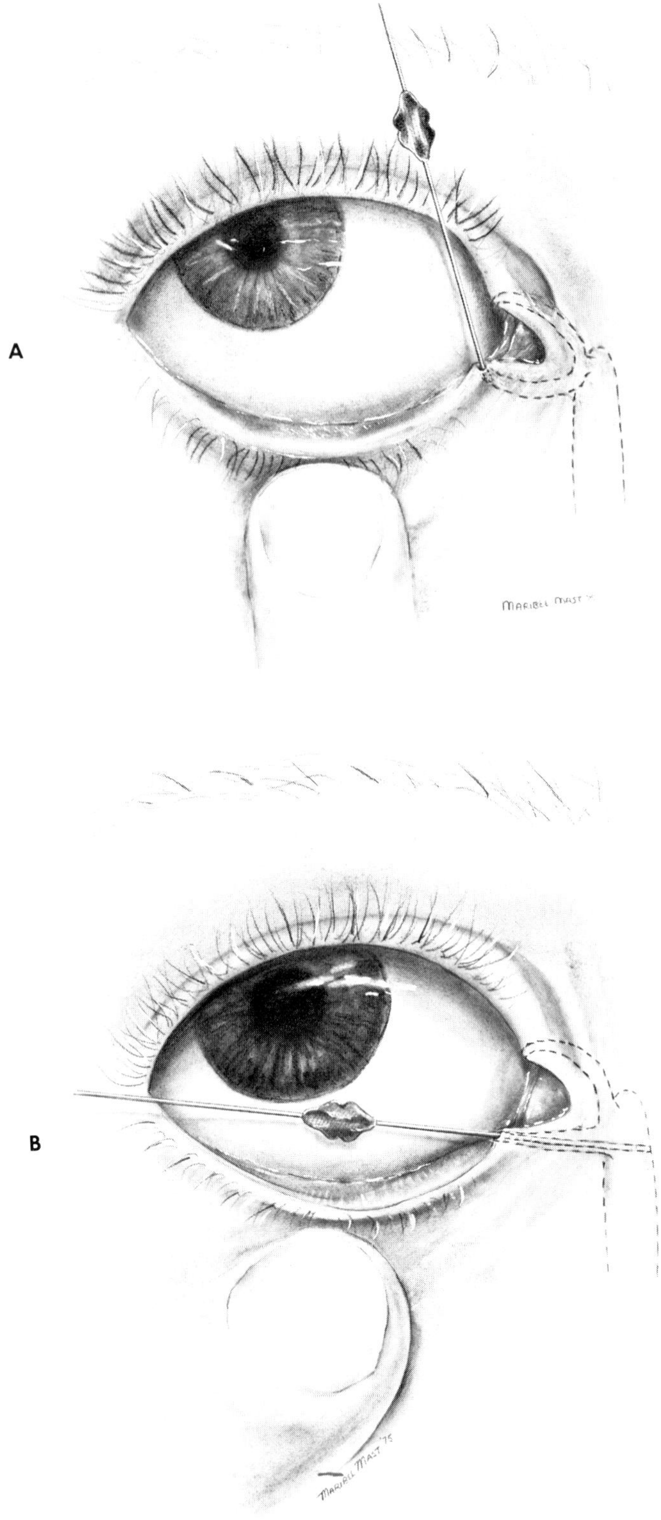

Fig. 4-2. Technique of probing. **A,** Bowman probe is passed in vertical direction, corresponding to vertical portion of canaliculus. Lid is moderately everted. **B,** Probe is brought into nearly horizontal position and gently directed toward nose while lid is pulled temporally; probe is stopped as soon as it touches medial wall of sac and its supporting bone.

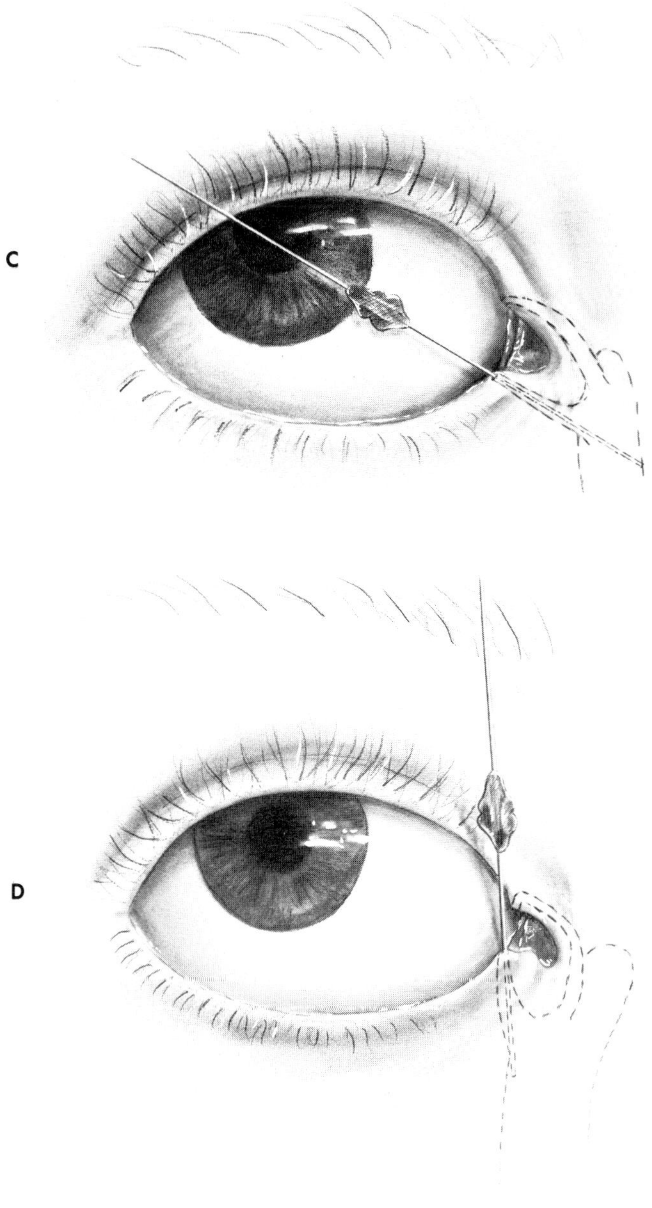

Fig. 4-2, cont'd. C, As probe is turned to vertical direction, temporal pull on lid is gradually released. **D,** Probe is pushed downward until lower extremity of nasolacrimal duct is penetrated.

who seem to have an osseous closure of the nasolacrimal duct or in whom the membranous occlusion has persisted until the child is too old for probing to effect a cure (after 12 to 24 months of age).

Injection of isotonic saline immediately following probing to test the effectiveness of the probing may save time, trouble, and embarrassment. With badly infected (acute or chronic) lacrimal sacs, probing occasionally may result in less favorable results. Administration of antibiotics for a few days prior to probing in these cases could produce a more favorable outcome.

Injury to the puncta, usually slitting, is an undesirable complication. Stenosis of the canaliculi is a serious complication. Both are the result of unnecessary trauma. Unintentional infiltration of soft tissues seldom causes a problem.

Technique. In most infants less than 6 months old, this can be performed satisfactorily as an office procedure. Administration of sedatives may facilitate the procedure, especially if the patient is past 5 or 6 months of age. Instillation of a topical anesthetic such as 0.5% proparacaine hydrochloride into the conjunctival sac may minimize the discomfort.

Satisfactory and safe preoperative preparation is provided by the following combination (doses for 10-kg patient): meperidine (Demerol), 25 mg; chlorpromazine (Thorazine), 6 mg; and promethazine (Phenergan), 6 mg.

Two assistants are usually needed to steady the infant who has been securely mummified in a sheet. A good light is essential. The parents are less disturbed if they are out of hearing distance. Because damage to the upper canaliculus is less serious than damage to the lower, it is preferable to probe through the upper. If this fails, the operator should immediately probe through the lower.

The punctal dilator is gently passed into the punctum in a vertical direction, dilating the punctum just sufficiently to allow a no. 0 or, at the largest, a no. 1 Bowman probe to enter. The probe is greased with any available ophthalmic ointment. When probing through the lower canaliculus, the probe is passed vertically for a millimeter or so (Fig. 4-2, *A*). The lid is pulled temporally, and the probe is then directed toward the nose (Fig. 4-2, *B*) until it is felt to meet the nasal wall of the lacrimal sac. While held snugly against the nasal wall of the sac (Fig. 4-2, *C*) the probe is brought to a near-vertical position (during this maneuver the tension on the lid temporally is gradually relaxed) and then gently guided inferiorly through the nasolacrimal duct (Fig. 4-2, *D*). A "popping" is often felt or even heard as the occluding membrane is ruptured.

Probing through the upper canaliculus is somewhat similar to probing through the lower except that the probe passes through this canaliculus in a direction midway between horizontal and vertical. After the probe enters the lacrimal sac, it is turned to a nearly vertical direction to pass through the nasolacrimal duct. If much force is required in the probing, the chances are that the probe is not directed in the proper direction.

Isotonic saline should be instilled immediately after probing (Fig. 4-3). If

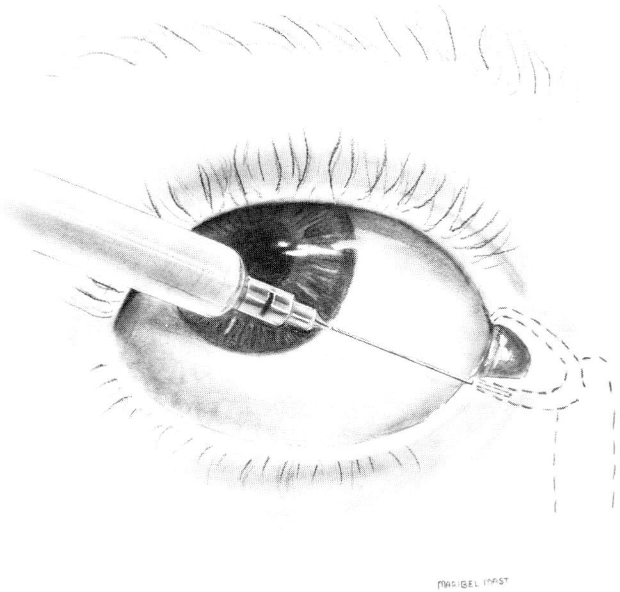

Fig. 4-3. Isotonic saline stained with a few drops of fluorescein is used to irrigate after probing. Irrigation determines if patency has been established and also cleanses sac and nasolacrimal duct of mucopus and other debris.

this enters the nose freely, the probing is likely to have been successful. Addition of a drop or two of dye such as fluorescein to the saline used for irrigation aids in detecting fluid exiting through the nasolacrimal duct. This is especially true if the probing is done under general anesthesia and the anesthesiologist is looking to see if the irrigating fluid enters the throat. If the fluid does not run freely into the nose, probing should be repeated immediately. If the first probing was through the upper canaliculus, probing through the lower may be tried, or vice versa. In some instances the nasolacrimal duct may be opened by lavage through the lower punctum while a punctum dilator is used to occlude the upper punctum (Fig. 4-4). This should be tried if probing has been unsuccessful. Care should be taken not to inject under too much pressure.

Light general anesthesia may be used (1) in patients past the age of 6 months, (2) when probing without general anesthesia has proved unsatisfactory, (3) when a dacryocystogram is indicated and cannot be done under sedation alone, or (4) when the ophthalmologist thinks it can be more successful, regardless of other considerations.

Difficult cases

If probing fails to effect a cure after attempts on two or three occasions in the favorable age group (under 6 months of age or even under 12 months), it

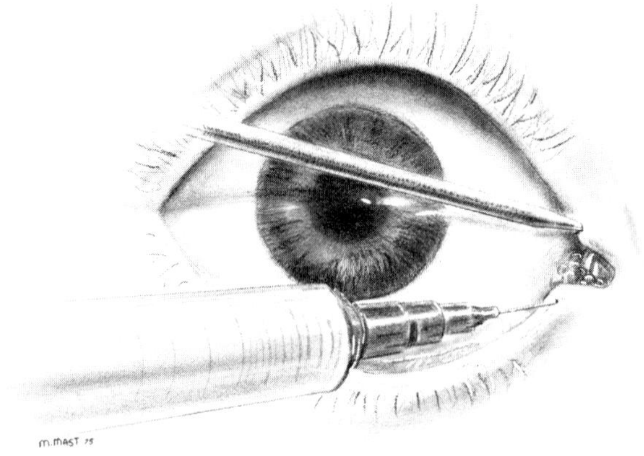

Fig. 4-4. Punctum dilator occluding upper punctum while isotonic saline is injected into lower canaliculus under mild pressure.

probably is wise for the ophthalmologist to refer the patient to a colleague for another probing. It is rare (possibly in less than 1% of infants under 6 months of age) that probing will not be successful, and these patients may have a congenital osseous obstruction of the nasolacrimal duct rather than a membranous one.

If probing is unsuccessful, a dacryocystogram may be helpful (see Chapter 8). The quality of the roentgenogram is often better if the injection of contrast medium is performed near the x-ray equipment and the roentgenogram taken immediately afterward. Sedation (see above) often will enable this technique to be carried out satisfactorily. If not, an anteroposterior view may be taken with the patient on the operating table under light general anesthesia. First, the lacrimal sacs are irrigated with isotonic saline to wash out as much of the contents as possible. Vigorous massage over the sacs will empty them of saline. Contrast medium is then gently injected bilaterally with the patient's head lowered sufficiently to prevent the fluid from entering the lungs if one of the sides is patent. In most instances the roentgenograms can be developed in the operating suite while the child is kept under light anesthesia so that further procedures can be carried out immediately if necessary. If further procedures are carried out, immediate postoperative dacryocystograms may be desirable.

In a few instances in which success seems doubtful from probing alone—especially when, after probing in older children, fluid can be lavaged into the nose only with difficulty—it may be helpful to inject some liquified (by warming) antibiotic-steroid ophthalmic ointment into the lacrimal sac under mild pressure from a 2-ml syringe fitted with a lacrimal cannula. Injection of long-acting penicillin, especially if much infection is present, may temporarily lessen

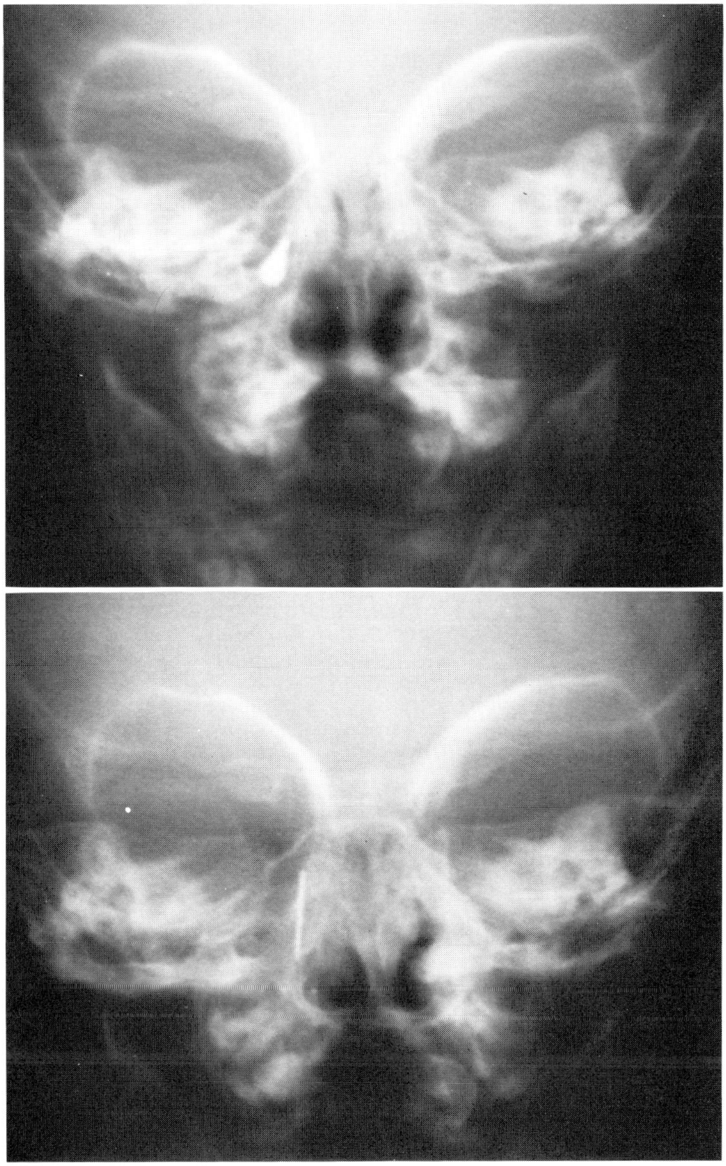

Fig. 4-5. Infant had undergone repeated unsuccessful probings. *Top,* Dacryocystogram before insertion of stainless steel canalicular rod. *Bottom,* Rod in place.

the infection and enhance the chances that probing and other procedures may effect a cure.

The use of a stainless steel canalicular rod similar to the one used to repair freshly severed canaliculi will often effect a cure when all other measures, short of an external dacryocystorhinostomy, fail. The 14-mm-long rod is preferable to the 12-mm one. General anesthesia is necessary. If the operator is convinced that failure is almost certain after the measures described above have been carried out (many of these young patients may already have undergone numerous probings over a period of weeks or months), a 14-mm-long stainless steel canalicular rod is gently passed into the upper canaliculus until only the 4-0 silk that is swaged on one end lies outside the upper punctum. The rod can easily be felt through the soft tissues. The operator cautiously "milks" the rod in a downward direction until the rod can be felt only barely or not at all (Fig. 4-5). It is preferable to take a roentgenogram immediately after the rod is inserted, to be sure that it is in proper position before it is anchored. With a curved needle threaded into it, the suture exiting from the upper punctum is anchored as described for repair of freshly severed canaliculi. The rod is removed in 3 to 4 weeks.

Instillation of a small amount of liquified antibiotic-steroid ointment into the canaliculi and intramuscular injection of long-acting penicillin may be helpful adjunctive procedures.

This method should be used carefully. I have limited this technique to those 2 years of age or younger. The parents should be warned that there are unfavorable cases, and cure may not occur. However, when the procedure is successful—as it is in about 75% of cases—the patient is spared a major operation at a later date. There is the rare possibility that the 4-0 suture will pull loose from the rod. In this case the patient is no worse off. The rod can be removed at external dacryocystorhinostomy performed when the patient is about 3 years old.

ANOMALIES OF LACRIMAL DRAINAGE SYSTEM

Congenital anomalies involving the canaliculi and puncta are fairly common. Many of these anomalies are asymptomatic and often go unrecognized. The upper canaliculus develops directly from the upper end of the column of solid epithelial cells destined to form the entire lacrimal drainage channel. The lower canaliculus is an offshoot of the precursor of the upper canaliculus. This probably explains why congenital anomalies of the lower canaliculus are more frequent.

Membranous closure of punctum

This anomaly has much in common with congenital stenosis of the nasolacrimal duct. Indeed, both conditions may be present in the same patient. Epiphora is the only symptom. A thin, dimpled membrane occludes the punctum. This membrane is easily ruptured with a punctum dilator. The newly opened

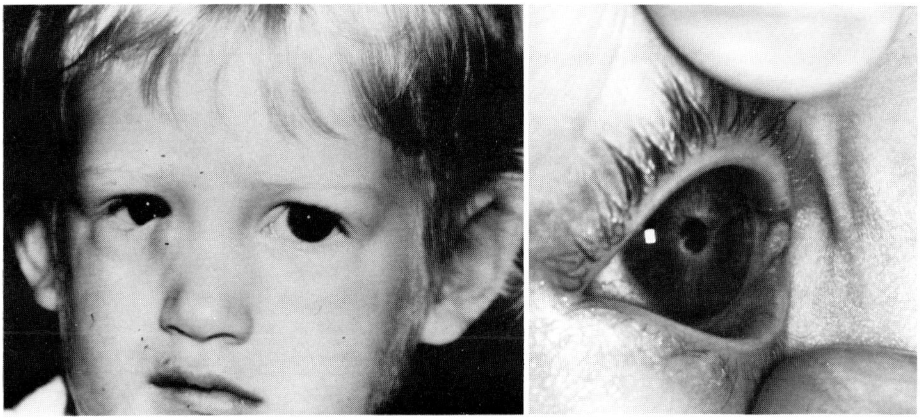

Fig. 4-6. Congenital occlusion of canaliculi and nasolacrimal duct on patient's right. Patient also had congenital hypoplasia of right optic nerve and imperforate anus. *Left,* Lacrimal sac is enormously enlarged and filled with mucus. *Right,* Congenital absence of the lower punctum and atresia of upper canaliculus.

punctum should be irrigated immediately with isotonic saline. If the nasolacrimal duct is occluded, it should be probed and the irrigation repeated. This condition is uncommon, but it is easily recognized. I have seen the condition only in the young. Effective treatment takes only a few moments.

Occlusion of punctum and canaliculus

In my experience this condition (Fig. 4-6) has been somewhat more common than the simple membrane occlusion of the punctum just described. The condition may be present in only one or two of the canaliculi or in all of them. The lower canaliculus is most commonly involved.

In older patients it may be impossible to distinguish congenital from acquired atresia of the punctum and canaliculus. A history of epiphora since birth is supportive evidence of congenital origin. Epiphora is the principal symptom. Some irritation may occur from stagnation of tears. Blurred vision due to excess tears may be very annoying, especially in cold, windy weather. On occasion the excess tears in the conjunctival sac interfere with the patient's activities.

When congenital occlusion involves the canaliculus as well as the punctum, treatment is usually difficult. In one case a 22-year-old dental student had tolerated his tearing until he reached the stage in dental school at which he had to work with his head bent forward. When he did this, tears dripped onto the patient's face—clearly an unhappy situation. Fortunately, the lower canaliculi were occluded only in the temporal 4 mm or so, and fashioning new puncta (more nasally than normal) for the patent nasal portion of the canaliculi relieved the epiphora.

In contrast to the ease in recognizing the punctal area when only a membranous occlusion exists, it usually is difficult to find the locus of the punctum when the canaliculus also is involved in the occlusion. If the upper punctum is visible, the examiner can estimate within a millimeter or two of where the lower punctum normally would be.

Correction of stenosis of punctum and canaliculus. The patient should be informed that the full extent of the problem cannot be determined preoperatively. An attempt should be made to establish patency in the lower canaliculi. An ample light and good magnification are essential. An attentive assistant to keep the field free of blood and, at times, to retract is a must.

The medial one third of the lower lid margin is injected with 2% lidocaine with a 30-gauge needle. With small straight scissors and a small-tooth forceps the dissection is begun at about where the punctum normally would be located. In the dissection to locate a patent punctum, care should be taken not to damage the outer edge of the lid to the extent that lid notching would result. The dissection is carried carefully toward the lacrimal sac. A patent part of the canaliculus usually is easily recognized and can be confirmed by injection of isotonic saline (from a syringe having a lacrimal tip) into the apparent canalicular opening. If the fluid enters the nose, a permanent punctum with a round opening is established. It is important that tissue be removed as far inferiorly (toward the lower cul-de-sac) as possible and also enough temporally to the opening so that tear drainage occurs and subsequent closure would be unlikely. If possible, the patient should be observed for several weeks or months.

Results of this procedure usually are satisfactory if the stenosis involves no more than the temporal 4 mm or so of the canaliculus. Greater nasal involvement compounds the difficulty. If no canaliculus can be found, one of the procedures that will bypass the canaliculus should be used (see Chapter 10).

There are other methods for locating the patent portion of the canaliculus. Jones[4] described opening the lacrimal sac and passing a no. 0 or 1 probe retrogradely through the common punctum into the canaliculus toward the external punctum. If there is a patent portion of the canaliculus, it can be seen by slitting along the conjunctival side of the margin of the eyelid until the probe is reached.

In LaPiana's[5] method the extent of the canalicular stenosis is determined by injecting methylene blue into the lacrimal sac. First, the skin along the anterior lacrimal crest is infiltrated with 2% lidocaine. A 27-gauge needle is inserted percutaneously until the floor of the lacrimal fossa is felt and then is withdrawn slightly. Methylene blue is injected into the sac while pressure is exerted over the inferior portion of the sac. A column of blue dye can be seen traversing patent canaliculi. A no. 11 Bard-Parker knife is used to incise the conjunctiva at the point reached by the dye. A circular ostium is fashioned in the canaliculus.

Supernumerary puncta and canaliculi

These are surprisingly common in occurrence but fortunately are usually asymptomatic, although epiphora has been reported in a few cases. They usu-

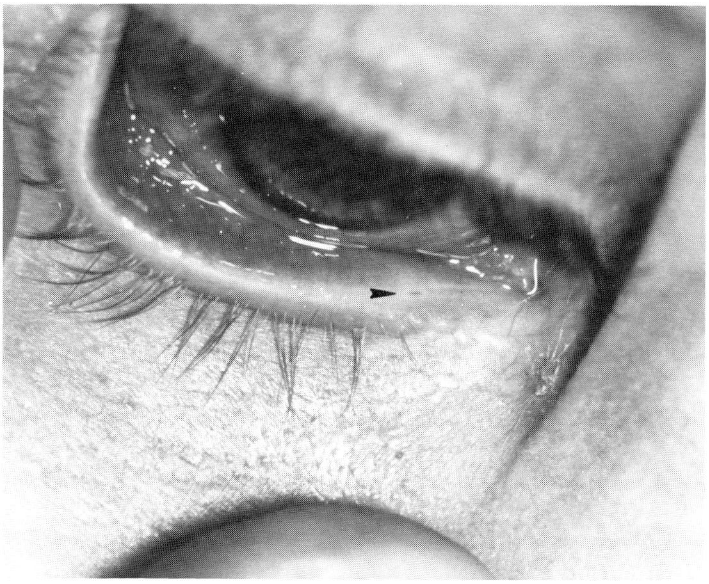

Fig. 4-7. Slit-shaped, small punctum *(arrow)*. Tissue around punctum and along lid margin to near the inner canthus was paper thin. Patient had had constant epiphora since birth.

ally occur on the lower lid and are not discovered by the examiner unless the medial portion of the lid is everted. The lid may have as many as three or four extra puncta but most often only one accessory punctum is present.

An accessory punctum may empty into the normal canaliculus, into an accessory canaliculus that may end blindly, or rarely, into the lacrimal sac separately from the normal canaliculus. Fig. 4-7 is from a case in which the patient had an abnormal punctum and patent canaliculus with constant epiphora. The punctum, a paper-thin slit, emptied into a patent canaliculus whose superior (lid) margin also apeared paper thin. A no. 0 Bowman probe passed into the canaliculus could be seen almost as easily as through slightly clouded glass. The epiphora apparently resulted from the absence of muscle to close the punctum on closure of the eyelids. The movement of the punctum nasally seemed mildly limited on eye closure. Making the punctum open more medially seemed to relieve the symptoms partially at the time, but we cannot be sure until there has been prolonged follow-up with fluorescein and Schirmer tests.

Occasionally, a mild, deforming, asymptomatic, congenital anomaly will be associated with the lacrimal drainage system. In one such case a small child had a teatlike deformity at the site of the upper punctum (Fig. 4-8).

Fistula

Congenital fistulas are not common, but when they are present and drain many tears onto the skin, considerable discomfort ensues. In some patients, tears

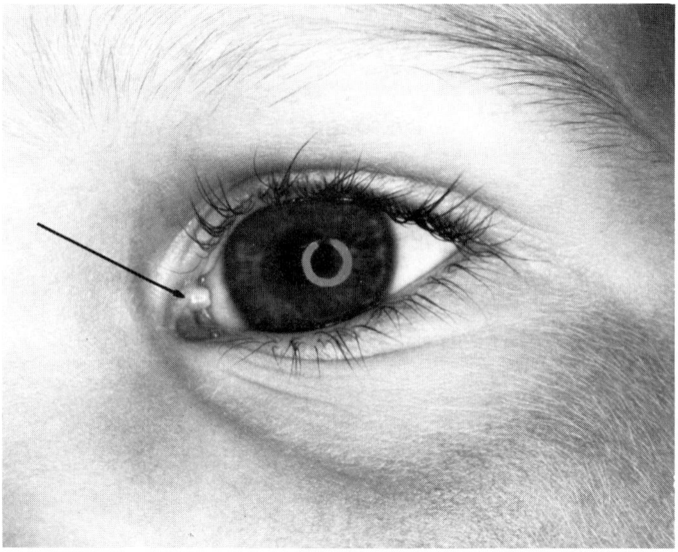

Fig. 4-8. Congenital teatlike deformity at site of upper punctum in child. Patient had no symptoms.

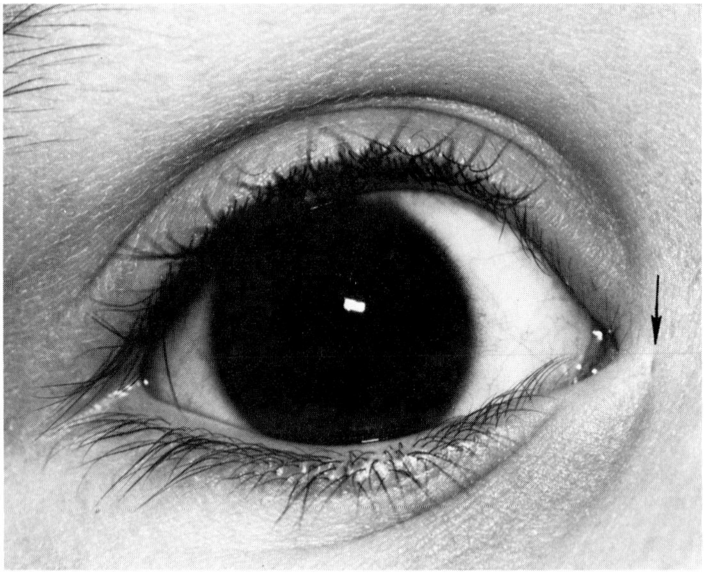

Fig. 4-9. Small congenital lacrimal fistula in 1½-year-old boy. Tears flowed through fistula when pressure was exerted on sac area. No spontaneous drainage was apparent. Impossible to determine exact origin of fistula by appearance. It could be from common canaliculus, lower canaliculus, or lacrimal sac.

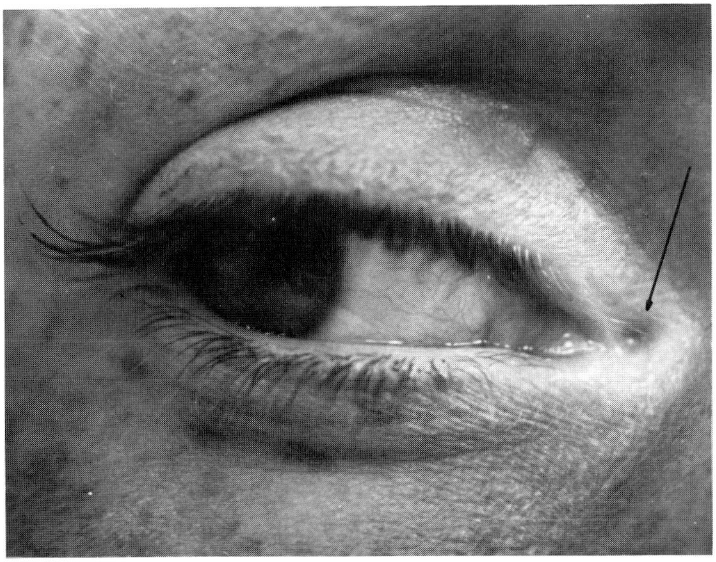

Fig. 4-10. Congenital fistula of upper canaliculus or common canaliculus.

do not exit through the fistula unless pressure is placed on the sac area (Fig. 4-9). The exact origin of a congenital fistula of the lacrimal system is impossible to determine with certainty from the appearance because many occur in the inner canthal region (Fig. 4-10).

A fistula originating in the lacrimal sac (Fig. 4-11) is not difficult to diagnose. If the sac is infected, mucopus can be expressed; otherwise, clear tears are evident. Congenital fistulas of the canaliculi are exceedingly rare. Congenital diverticula, if they occur, most likely would go unrecognized. Infections of the canaliculi that cause concretion may develop because of congenital diverticula.

Fistulas from the lacrimal gland are exceedingly rare; in most cases the fistula opens into the outer aspect of the upper lid at about the level of the superior margin of the tarsus, although in one case it opened temporally to the lateral canthus.

Treatment may be transplantation of the fistula into the upper conjunctival cul-de-sac. If that fails, the tract could be cauterized or the fistula could be excised along with that portion of the lacrimal gland from which the fistula originated.

Eversion (ectopic)

Congenital eversion (ectopia of the punctum) is rare. The punctum may be seen without eversion of the lid (Fig. 4-12). Unless the diagnosis is made when the patient is young, distinguishing congenital from acquired eversion may be impossible. Epiphora is the only symptom. Correction is the same as that for acquired ectropion.

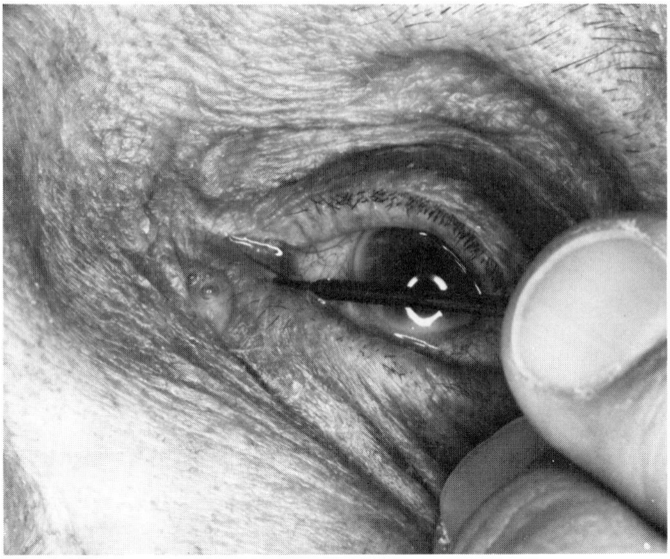

Fig. 4-11. Lacrimal sac fistula. Mucopus was easily expressed.

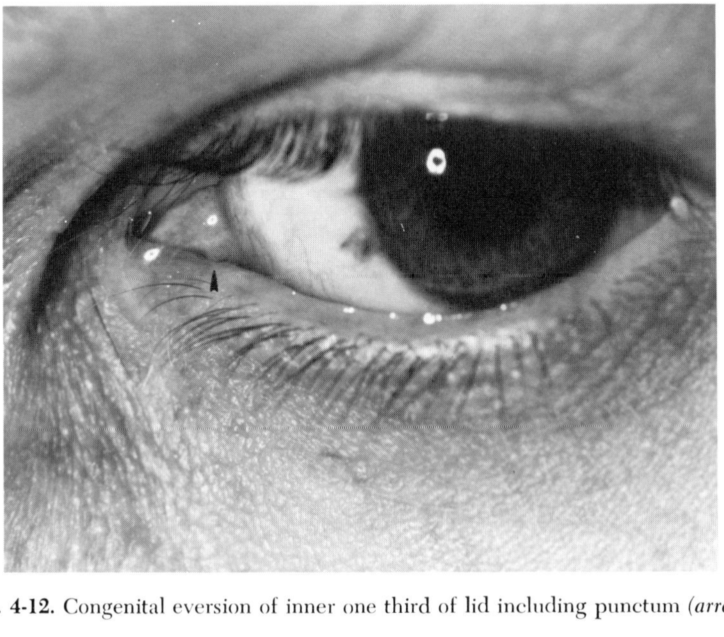

Fig. 4-12. Congenital eversion of inner one third of lid including punctum *(arrow)*.

ANOMALIES OF THE LACRIMAL GLAND

The lacrimal gland develops from ingrowth of epithelium from the conjunctiva of the outer portion of the upper fornix. Congenital anomalies are relatively rare.

Aberrant and ectopic lacrimal gland anomalies

Confusion exists in the terminology. Gördüren[2] described the difference as follows: in the aberrant forms the main lacrimal gland is in its place, and the other gland is additional; in ectopia, the original lacrimal gland is considered to be displaced. Ectopia is not as rare as aberrant tissue.

Green and Zimmerman[3] apparently considered "aberrant lacrimal gland" and "ectopic lacrimal gland" as synonymous in their review of 35 cases. The cornea was involved in 10 of 18 cases with choristomatous lesions (lesions that clinically produce tumefaction). Ectopic lacrimal gland tissue was within the eye in one case. Ectopic or aberrant gland tissue has been found deep in the orbit, causing proptosis. Such tissue can occur at other ocular locations.

Alacrima

Congenital alacrima is a rare condition that is most commonly seen in familial dysautonomia (commonly called Riley-Day syndrome). The condition is frequently seen in siblings and in persons of Jewish extraction. The disorder is manifested by specific malfunctions of the central nervous system, especially of autonomic function. Defective lacrimation is one of the many serious manifestations of the disease. The lacrimal gland is normal histologically and will produce tears when stimulated by methacholine eye drops used topically. Corneal sensitivity is often decreased or absent. Corneal ulcers occur commonly. Unilateral congenital alacrima is exceedingly rare.

REFERENCES

1. Beckerman, B. L.: Lacrimal anomalies in anhidrotic ectodermal dysplasia, Am J Ophthalmol 75:728-730, 1973.
2. Gördüren, S.: Aberrant lacrimal gland associated with other congenital abnormalities, Br J Ophthalmol 46:277-280, 1962.
3. Green, W. R., and Zimmerman, L. E.: Ectopic lacrimal gland tissue. Report of eight cases with orbital involvement, Arch Ophthalmol 78:318-327, 1967.
4. Jones, L. T.: The cure of epiphora due to canalicular disorders, trauma and surgical failures on the lacrimal passages, Trans Am Acad Ophthalmol Otolaryngol 66:506-524, 1962.
5. LaPiana, F. G.: Management of occult atretic lacrimal puncta, Am J Ophthalmol 74:332-333, 1972.
6. Turner, J. B.: A clinical review of congenital glaucoma, South Med J 64:1362-1365, 1971.

CHAPTER 5

Disorders of the canaliculi and eyelids

Epiphora can be defined as an abnormal overflow of tears onto the cheek due to defective tear drainage, usually as a result of an obstruction. This condition is common and can have a great variety of causes, many subtle.

Patience and time may be required for proper evaluation of these patients. Many of the tests described in Chapter 3 will be found useful. Some patients with severe epiphora may have an overproduction of tears that aggravates their defective drainage. Indeed, the irritation from the overflow of tears may create a vicious cycle—the inflammation caused by the excessive accumulation and overflow along with further irritation from excessive wiping of the eyelids will stimulate production of still more tears. This is especially annoying in those exposed to cold winds.

LACRIMAL CANALICULITIS

Lacrimal canaliculitis with concretions

This is a chronic infection, almost always limited to one canaliculus and typically slow in its onset and course. The usually mentioned infecting agent is a fungus. Von Graefe in 1854 was the first to recognize actinomyces as a causative organism.

Etiology. *Actinomyces israelii*, an anaerobic bacterium and not a fungus, is the organism most commonly responsible for the concretion-forming canaliculitis that is generally described as being due to fungi. (An archaic term, "streptothrix," that often is applied to this organism should be discarded.) Another bacterial genus whose members—aerobes—produce a similar clinical picture is *Nocardia*. Two aerobic fungi have been implicated, *Candida albicans*, a yeastlike fungus, and *Aspergillus niger*. There is no firm evidence as to how the organisms reach the canaliculus or what triggers the start of the infection. It has been postulated that a preexisting diverticulum of the involved canaliculus predisposes to development of infection.

Clinical findings. The onset usually is slow. One of my patients was free of

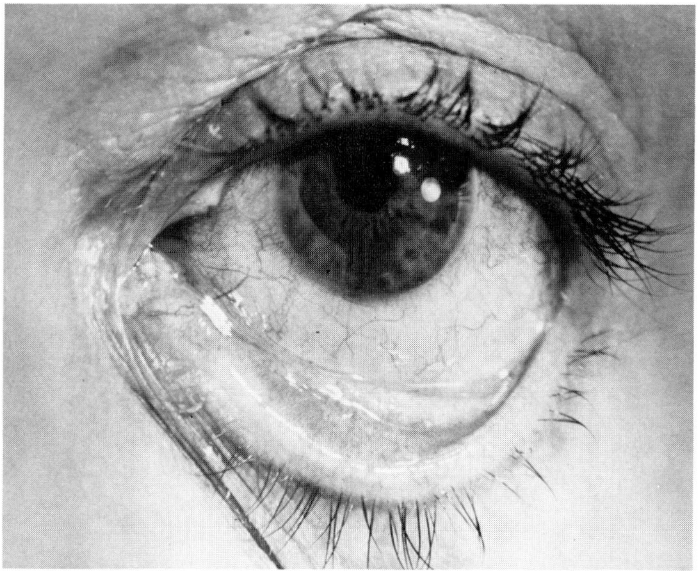

Fig. 5-1. Mild canaliculitis of lower lid. Signs and symptoms of inflammation developed in 6-week interval between office visits. A few concretions were removed from canaliculus.

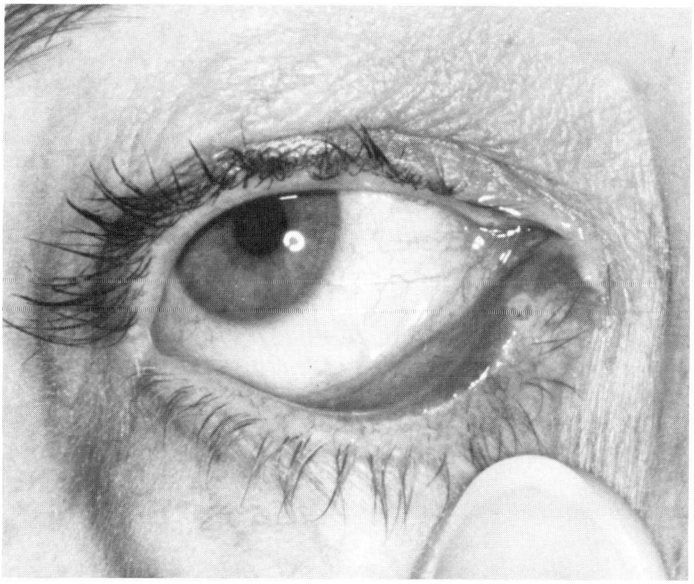

Fig. 5-2. Moderately severe canaliculitis with punctum having pouting appearance. Pus was easily expressed. A large number of concretions were removed.

any symptoms suggestive of canaliculitis at examination, but 6 weeks later mild but easily recognized edema and infection of the punctal area of a lid had developed (Fig. 5-1). A few concretions were present within the canaliculus. Unless the ophthalmologist keeps in mind that canaliculitis is one cause of chronic unilateral inflammation of the eye, the condition will go unrecognized. The condition occurs more often in women and more often in the lower canaliculus.

The early symptoms are mild injection, slight edema of the area of the involved canaliculus, and epiphora. As time passes, the swelling and irritation increase and the conjunctivitis, primarily limited to the inner canthal region, becomes more extensive. The lid margin swelling, most marked at the involved punctum, increases, and the punctum assumes a pouting appearance with a mild ectropion (Fig. 5-2). Mild pressure on the involved canaliculus, especially if a glass rod is applied on the inner aspect of the lid, will cause pus (and occasionally a concretion) to extrude through the punctum.

Almost invariably, isotonic saline can be lavaged through the involved canaliculus into the nose prior to removal of the concretions. I have seen only two instances in which this was not the case: after removal of the concretions, saline could be irrigated into the nose in one of these patients; the other had a stenosis near the common canaliculus (Fig. 5-3).

Most patients with this type of canaliculitis are adults, most often middle-aged or older. I have seen one case in a 15-year-old girl who had a history of watering and tearing of her right eye "practically all of her life" (Fig. 5-4); the upper canaliculus was enormously dilated.

Treatment. Complete removal of concretions from the involved canaliculus is essential for cure. A small lacrimal probe can be passed through the punctum into the canaliculus. After the canalicular area is injected with a small amount of lidocaine, a 3- or 4-mm horizontal incision is made into the canaliculus just inside the lid margin. There is no advantage to carrying the incision laterally to include the punctum, although when this has been done epiphora has not persisted. Usually, the canaliculus is greatly dilated and filled with concretions. These can be picked out with small forceps. The canaliculus is thoroughly lavaged to make certain that all concretions have been removed. The incision is sutured with fine silk.

The original incision can be made through the punctum and the canaliculus opened medially just inside the lid margin, especially if the upper canaliculus is involved. I prefer to suture these incisions; others report no problem without suturing. There is probably no need to suture the upper canaliculus.

The common infecting organisms are sensitive to penicillin and other antibiotics, and the canaliculus may be irrigated with an antibiotic solution after the operation, but I have never seen a recurrence in cases in which this was not done.

Unless all the concretions are removed the canaliculitis will continue indefinitely. One woman operated on by me had had unilateral involvement of

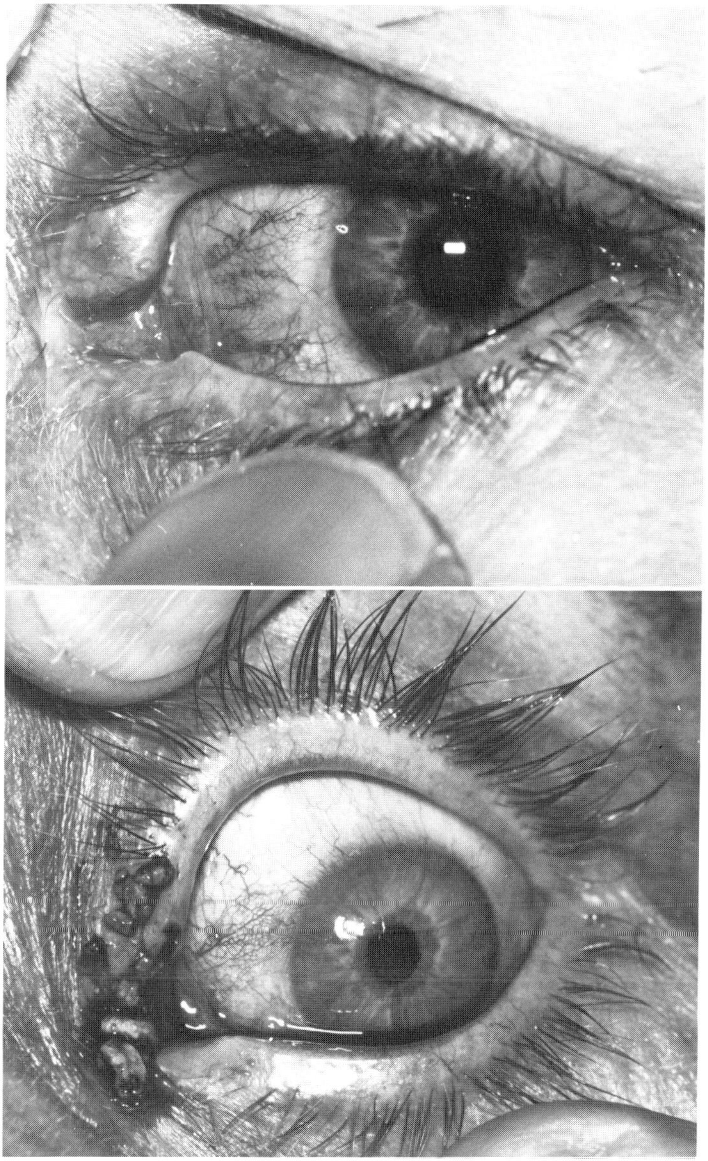

Fig. 5-3. Case of canaliculitis in which saline could not be irrigated into nose. *Top,* Pouting, edema, and dilatation of upper punctum. *Bottom,* Large number of concretions removed after incision of upper punctum. Morphologically they suggest *Streptomyces* or *Nocardia.* Upper canaliculus was found to be stenosed near upper punctum.

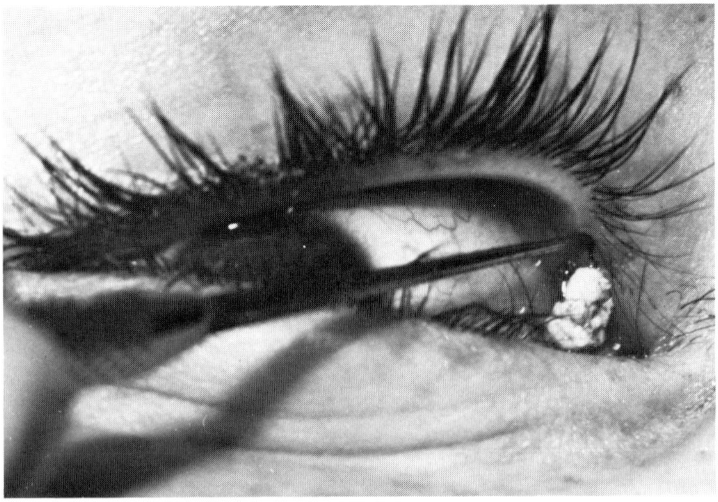

Fig. 5-4. Canaliculitis in 15-year-old girl with history of long-standing epiphora and irritation of right eye. Concretions shown here represented about half the amount removed. Anaerobic culture showed a gram-positive bacillus identified biochemically as *Actinomyces naeslundii.*

both canaliculi for more than 20 years. The infecting organism or the accompanying secondary infection may respond temporarily to antibiotic or other treatment, but the disease follows a course of remissions and exacerbations until the concretions are completely removed.

Miscellaneous lacrimal canaliculitis

Undoubtedly, lacrimal canaliculitis may result from any of a large variety of causes. Some degree of canalicular involvement may occur with acute or chronic conjunctivitis. Most of these cases clear spontaneously, and the condition is unrecognized.

Canalicular involvement may occur with a number of other ocular disorders, for example, trachoma, pemphigus, herpes simplex, herpes zoster, and Stevens-Johnson syndrome. Treatment of the primary ocular condition at an early stage (early trachoma, for example) may prevent total stenosis of the canaliculus. Pneumococci, staphylococci, gonococci, and other commonplace bacteria on rare occasions have been reported as causing canaliculitis.

An abscess may occur in a canaliculus that is markedly dilated when first seen. The punctum was completely stenosed in one case that I treated. No organism could be cultured.

Kalt and Kalt[2] demonstrated that inflammation due to infectious conjunctivitis occasionally may spread to cause a follicular canaliculitis, especially in old persons. A massive subepithelial infiltration of lymphocytes with plasma cells collects as follicles around the canaliculi, especially at their junctions with the sac. The epithelium may remain nearly normal. Epiphora is the principal

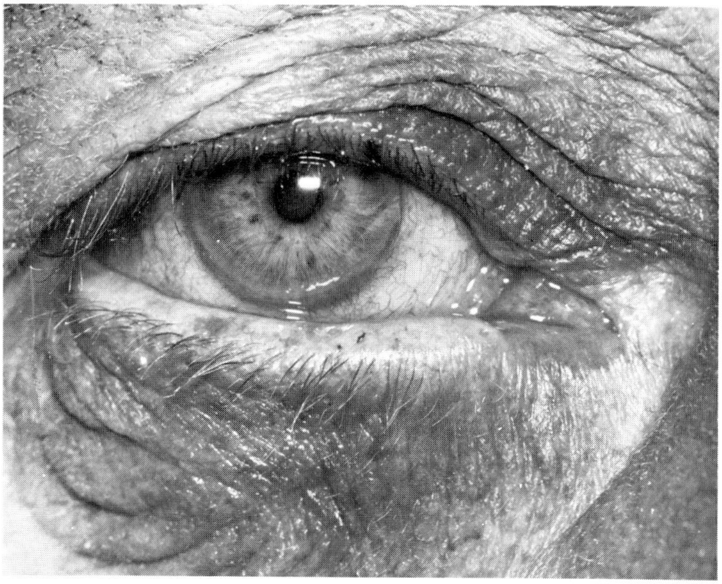

Fig. 5-5. Mild ectropion. Tears cannot enter lower punctum because of eversion.

symptom. This finding would adequately explain the comparatively large number of elderly persons who develop unexplained epiphora, usually bilaterally.

In some cases, when saline is irrigated through the lower canaliculus, some will enter the nose, and some will exit through the upper punctum or vice versa. In other cases, when saline is irrigated through one canaliculus, all the fluid will exit from the other ipsilateral canaliculus, indicating stenosis of the ampullary portion of the common canaliculus.

DISORDERS OF THE EYELIDS

The puncta, especially the lower puncta, must be examined with the utmost care. What might appear to be insignificant or totally missed by the examiner may be the principal if not the only cause for the epiphora.

Ectropion of lid involving lower punctum

Diagnosis. This condition is seen more frequently in older persons, in whom it develops spontaneously. In the mildest form of the condition the lower punctum will be pointing vertically and can be visualized without everting the lower lid (Fig. 5-5). (Normally, the lower punctum is pointing in a more posterior direction, hugging the eyeball no matter what direction the eye turns.) Upon close observation, preferably under a slitlamp, it will be seen that no tears can enter these puncta. The inability of tears to enter the punctum can be shown by instilling fluorescein into the conjunctival sacs—the stained tears will stop 1 mm or so short of reaching the punctum.

Ectropion can vary from the very mild as just described to the severe. All

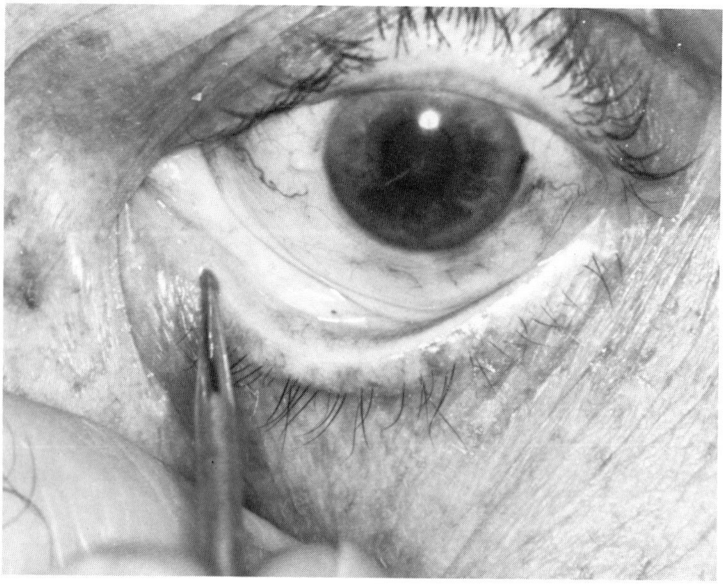

Fig. 5-6. Punctum is dilated prior to irrigation with saline to determine patency.

cases have one thing in common: spontaneous drainage of tears does not occur through the everted punctum.

Treatment. Common sense should prevail in deciding what treatment, if any, is indicated. In many elderly persons with mildly atonic lids the punctum may turn outward to the point that spontaneous drainage through it is impossible. If the accompanying epiphora is mild to moderate, the patient may prefer to tolerate the annoyance. These patients should be advised to wipe their eyes only in an upward direction. Wiping in a downward direction would tend to aggravate their ectropion.

Before any type of surgical procedure is attempted to correct the epiphora, it is well to know the patient's approximate rate of tear production. A few elderly persons, the weepy, emotional type, may secrete tears almost as fast as the Schirmer test will measure them, and their primary problem is excessive lacrimation rather than a lack of drainage. These patients are almost universally disappointed in their surgical results, regardless of how good the appearance may be. If surgical treatment is planned for this type of patient, the patient should be warned that the results may fall short of ideal. Removal of the palpebral lobe of the lacrimal gland in this type of patient offers an approximately 50% chance of appreciable relief. The danger of developing a dry eye by removal of the gland in these elderly weepy persons is highly improbable.

In mild ectropion, several procedures are useful if properly performed.

Three-snip procedure. The lid margin is injected with 2% lidocaine via a 30-gauge needle. The punctum is gently dilated (Fig. 5-6). Fluid is irrigated into

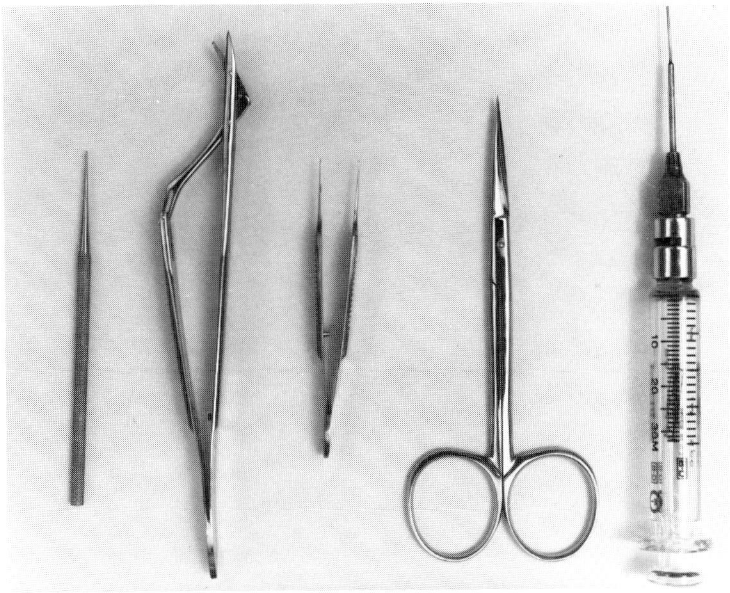

Fig. 5-7. Instruments used to perform three-snip operation.

the canaliculus to determine the patency of the remainder of the drainage system. A small, straight-pointed scissors (Fig. 5-7) is inserted into the punctum and directed medially for 2 to 3 mm along the conjunctival inner lid margin, and the first snip is made (Fig. 5-8, *top*). Then the blade of the same scissors is inserted at the nasal extremity of the first incision and directed downward and temporally for approximately 2 mm for the second snip (Fig. 5-8, *middle*). With one blade of the scissors inserted at the temporal end of the first incision and the scissors directed downward and nasally, the third snip is taken (Fig. 5-8, *bottom*). The most important consideration is directing the scissors in the second and third snips so that they will meet at the depth of the vertical portion of the canaliculus, which is about 2 mm. The new opening of the punctum will be round and in good position to permit tears to enter.

Holth punch. This accomplishes the same purpose as the classic three-snip operation. The first snip is made into the canaliculus about 2.5 mm along the lid margin, as shown in Fig. 5-8, *top*. By grasping the skin along the lid margin with a small-toothed forceps, the lid is pulled away from the direction of the Holth punch (2-mm width). The Holth punch is then directed toward the lower cul-de-sac (in the vertical portion of the canaliculus) for a depth of approximately 2 mm, and the blades are closed sharply (Fig. 5-9, *top*). A similar portion of tissue is removed as in the three-snip procedure. As before, the removal of tissue must be carried downward to the extremity of the vertical part of the canaliculus (Fig. 5-9, *bottom*). The results can be most gratifying if the procedure is performed correctly and when indicated. If the procedure is incor-

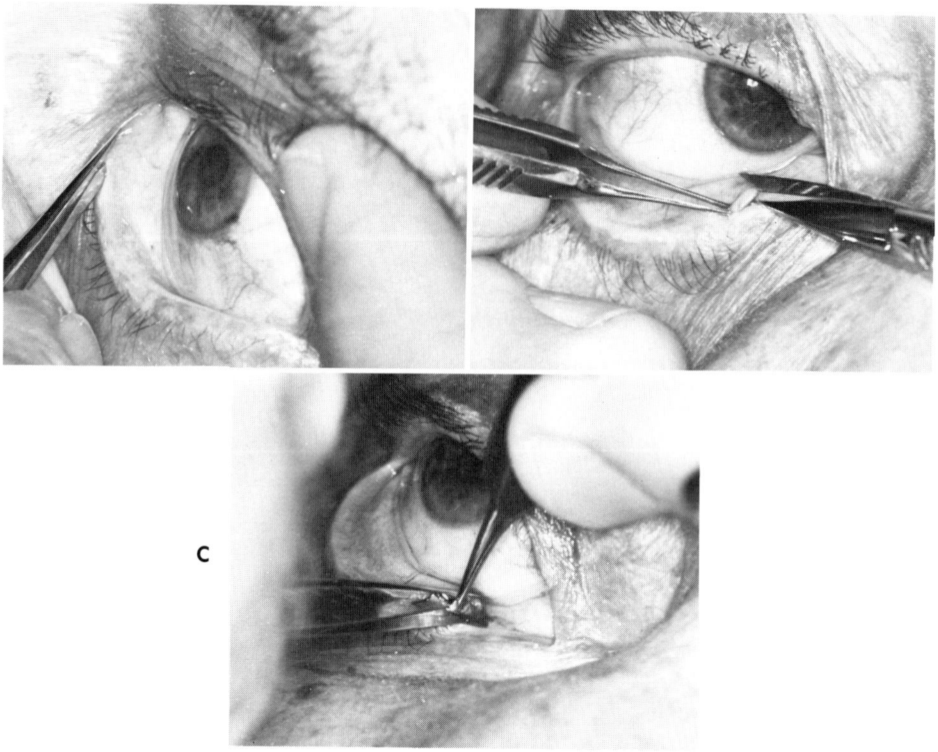
A B C

Fig. 5-8. Three-snip operation. **A,** First snip is in conjunctiva along lid margin, about 2 mm long. **B,** Second snip. Scissors, at nasal end of first incision, is directed temporally and downward to depth of vertical portion of canaliculus. **C,** Third snip. Scissors, at temporal end of first incision, is directed nasally and downward to depth of vertical portion of canaliculus. Removal of triangular portion of tissue produces round opening into canaliculus, nearer lower cul-de-sac.

rectly performed or performed without proper indications, it will give disappointing results. Fluorescein should enter the nose spontaneously, and most importantly, the patient should obtain relief.

Other procedures. The one-snip procedure is performed with just one snip on the conjunctival side of the punctum.

Application of a point cautery at multiple sites—through the palpebral conjunctiva, nasally, inferiorly, and temporally to the newly created canalicular opening (taking care not to apply the points too closely, thus damaging the operated area)—may decrease the ectropion to a minor degree.

Occasionally, a markedly enlarged caruncle will "push" the punctum outward enough to interfere with tear drainage (Fig. 5-10). Removal of about half or more of the caruncle may solve the problem.

Removal of a spindle-shaped piece of tissue from the inside of the lower lid is another easily performed procedure that is useful for treating mild-to-moderate ectropion involving the lower punctum. After injection of local anesthetic into

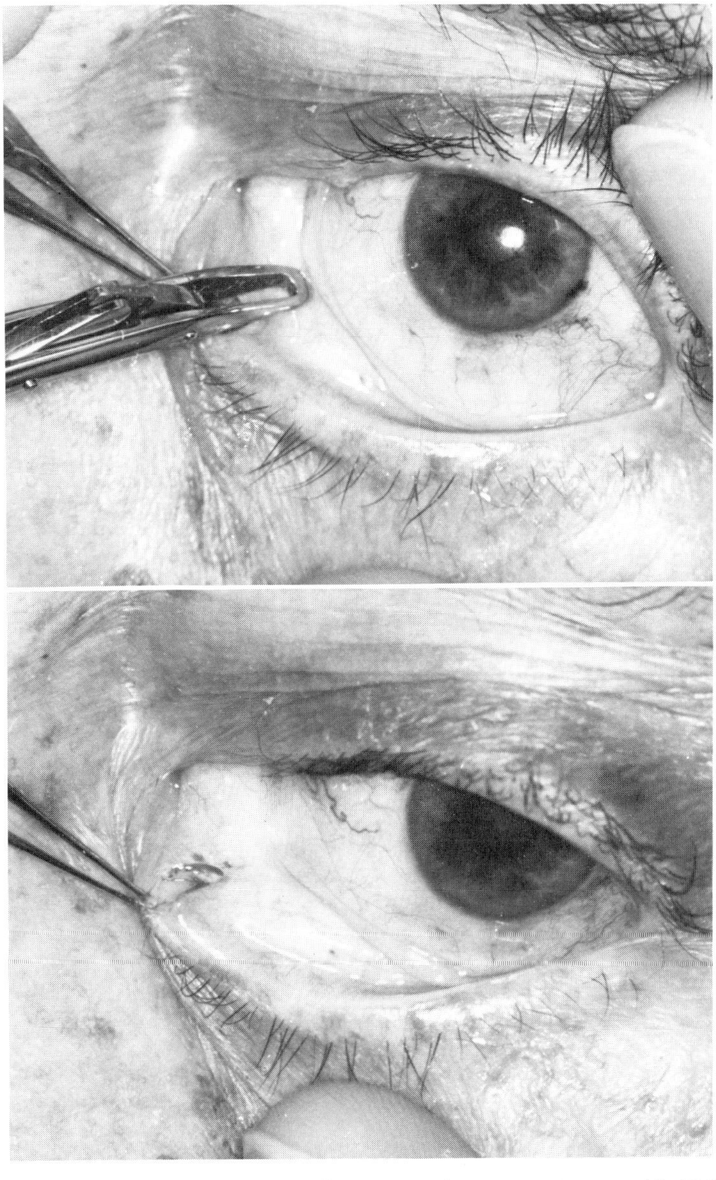

Fig. 5-9. Use of Holth punch. *Top,* After first snip with scissors, 2-mm-width Holth punch is placed so its blade will reach as far inferiorly as possible (2 mm). Toothed forceps is used to grasp lid margin and pull forward against Holth punch. *Bottom,* Oval opening into canaliculus after use of Holth punch. Opening is sufficiently wide (2 mm) and deep (2 mm) so as not to close but still drain tears.

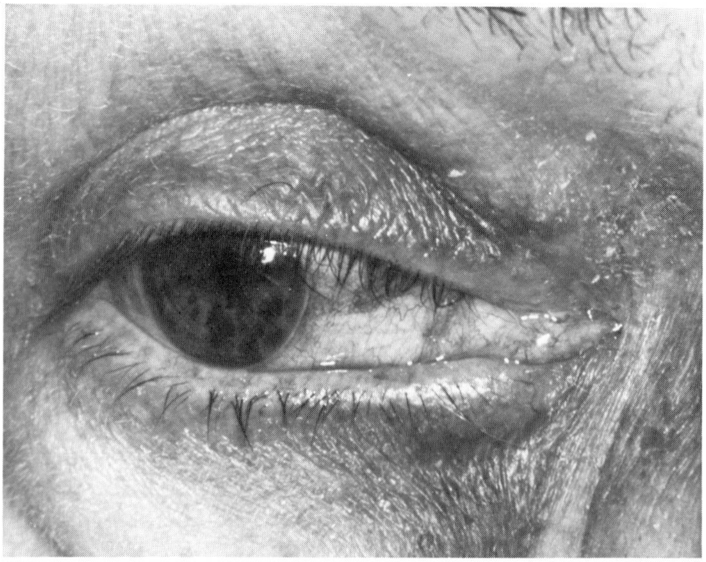

Fig. 5-10. Hypertrophied caruncle "pushing" punctum outward.

the lower lid, a large (15-mm width) chalazion clamp is clamped in position with the open end on the conjunctival side. The clamp end must be directed toward the lower end of the cul-de-sac and clamped tightly; otherwise, the clamp will slip (Fig. 5-11, *top*). A spindle-shaped outline is made in the palpebral conjunctiva held within the clamp (without the clamp, the tissues are most difficult to handle). The tissue removed in this spindle should extend from a point 2 mm from the lower punctum temporally for a distance of about 10 mm. The extremities of the spindle come to a point; at its center it should be 3 to 4 mm in width. After the conjunctival and subconjunctival tissues are excised with scissors and toothed forceps, three double-arm small sutures (such as 6-0 silk) are passed into one cut edge of the wound and across the wound to engage the suture in the cut edge of the opposite side. After all the sutures are placed (but not tied), the chalazion clamp is removed (Fig. 5-11, *bottom*). Removal of the clamp allows the wound edges to be approximated with the sutures.

Weakness of orbicularis oculi muscles

Epiphora due to weakness of the orbicularis oculi muscles is common. This may occur as a normal aging process, or its onset may be more dramatic as with paralysis of these muscles. With loss of tonicity of the orbicularis muscle, the lower punctum moves feebly (or not at all in total paralysis) during opening and closing of the eyelids. This weakness greatly reduces the pumping action in tear drainage. Also, the lower punctum is usually turned outward, away from contact with the tears.

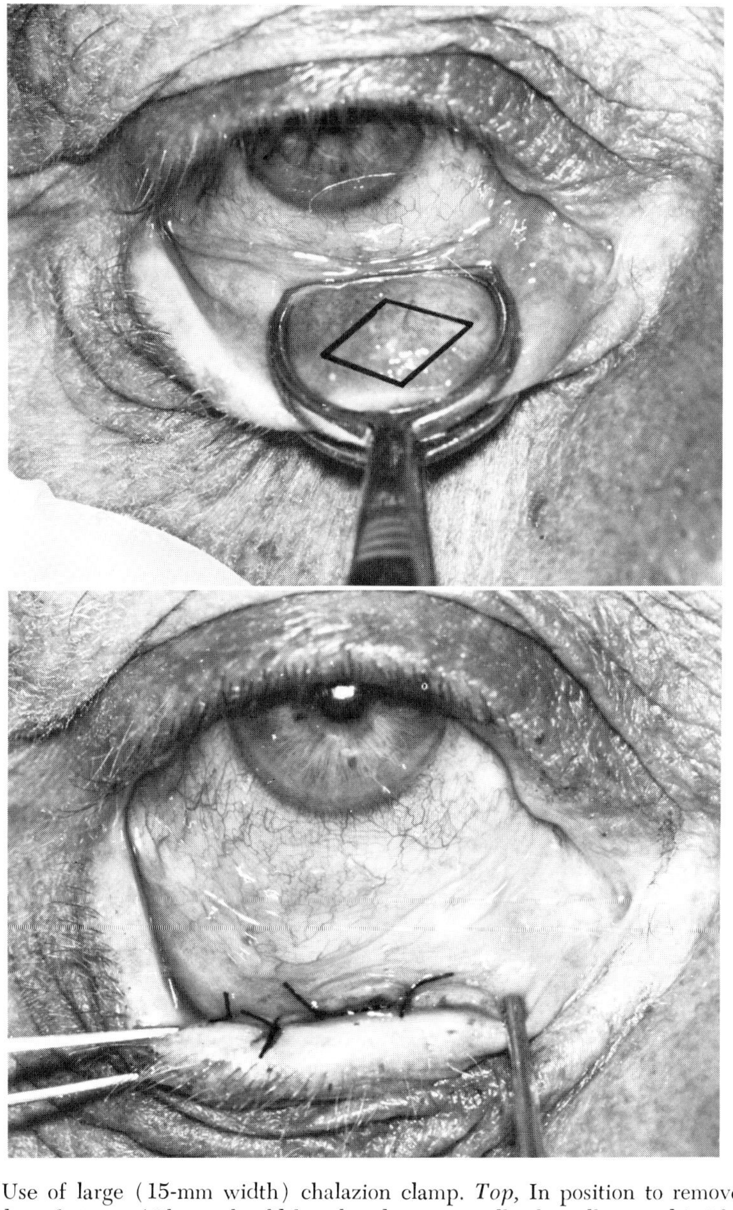

Fig. 5-11. Use of large (15-mm width) chalazion clamp. *Top,* In position to remove spindle-shaped wedge of tissue. (Clamp should be placed more nasally than illustrated.) After sutures are placed, clamp must be removed to permit tying of sutures to close wound. *Bottom,* Chalazion clamp removed and sutures tied.

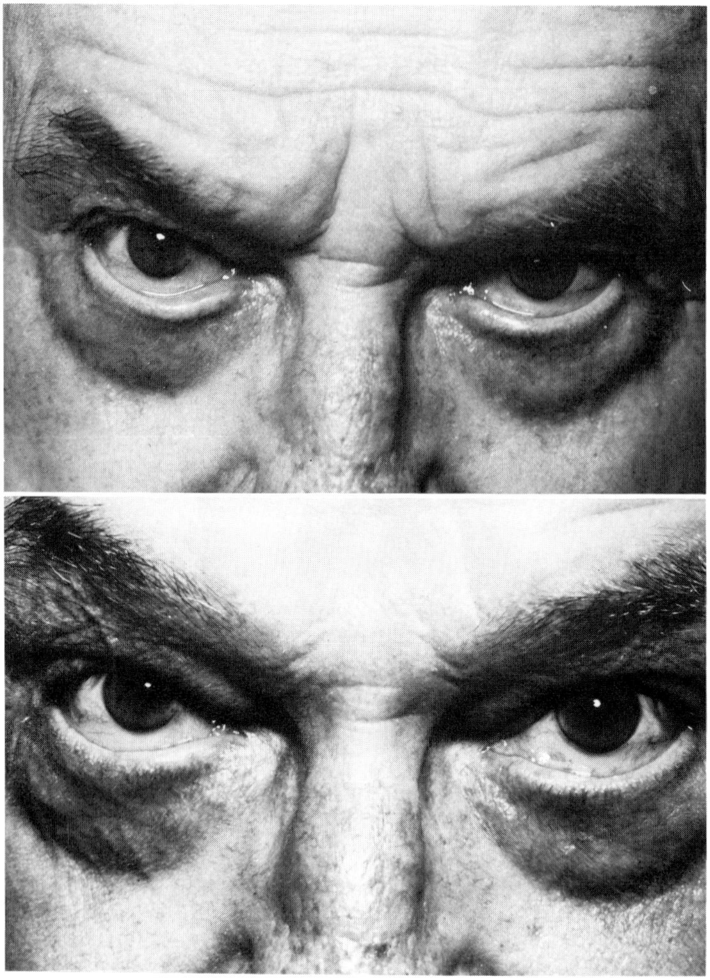

Fig. 5-12. Senile ectropion. *Top,* Preoperative appearance. (From Veirs, E. R.: The lacrimal system in clinical practice, Rochester, Minn., 1963, American Academy of Ophthalmology and Otolaryngology, p. 35.) *Bottom,* Appearance after Kuhnt-Szymanowski operation.

The results of treatment may not be ideal. Even if the punctum is altered so as to be in contact with the tear film, the weakness of the orbicularis muscles may result in epiphora. Jacobs[1] recommended exercise for the weak muscles. The patient is instructed to exercise three times a day by making a slow, sustained, winking movement or a straining visual effort 20 times; this regimen is followed for several months. In his experience the exercise did not benefit the elderly.

Senile ectropion (atonic)

Senile or atonic ectropion of considerable severity is usually seen in patients in their eighth decade or older. Its development is slow. Many patients are

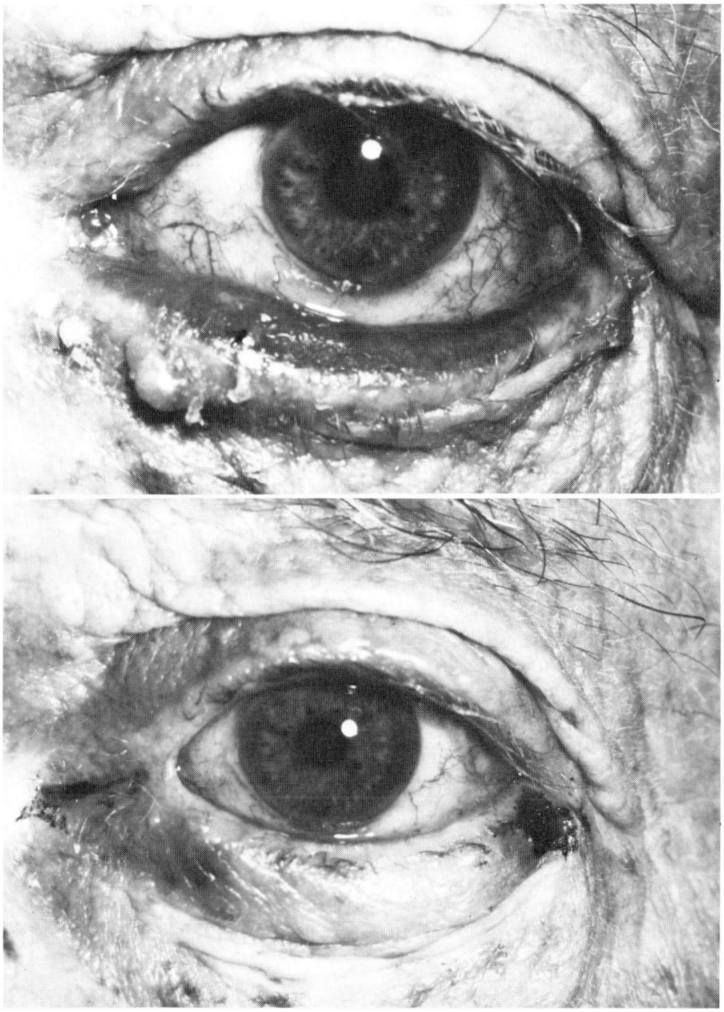

Fig. 5-13. Cicatricial ectropion. *Top,* Markedly irritated eye preoperatively. *Bottom,* After use of generous skin graft and tarsorrhaphy. Tarsorrhaphy can later be cut with lid holding in good position.

bothered little by epiphora or by the appearance and prefer to live with their condition. More of the lower part of their eyes and lower palpebral conjunctiva are exposed to irritation from wind, smog, and the like, resulting in increased reflex lacrimation. The Kuhnt-Szymanowski operation or some modification of this procedure offers good cosmetic as well as functional results (Fig. 5-12). The decrease in epiphora may be more a result of elimination of the eye irritation (which stimulates excess lacrimation) rather than of improvement in drainage.

Cicatricial ectropion

Cicatricial ectropion is commonly seen in persons with fair complexions and who experience long exposure to sunlight. (Many develop basal cell epitheliomas on the face, including the lower lids especially.) Trauma and burns are not infrequent causes. Overzealous surgery on the lower lid is another cause. Fig. 5-13 shows a severe cicatricial ectropion that developed from long exposure to the sun. If epiphora is decreased postoperatively in this type of patient, the credit probably belongs more to diminished irritation than to better tear drainage.

ACQUIRED STENOSIS

Acquired stenosis of punctum

Tears will drain adequately through a punctum whose opening is so small as to be difficult to see—this can be proved with the fluorescein dye test. The shape of the opening may vary: round, oval, or slit. However, when a punctum is closed physiologically but not stenosed, epiphora may occur.

The completely stenosed punctum cannot be opened without forcing adherent tissues apart. The puncta frequently diminish in size with age. Irritation from infection, eye medications, and trauma (for example, injuries or probing) may cause a cicatricial closure.

Patients who secrete few tears and have little epiphora (especially the elderly) may prefer to have no treatment. Locating the exact position of where the punctum belongs may not be simple. The lid margin may give no hint. Often, the punctal area will appear pale because of its diminished vascularity. If possible, one should estimate the distance from the inner canthus or from the location of the upper punctum. Injection of the lid margin with 2% lidocaine via a 30-gauge needle may be needed. Downward probing for a short distance with a sharp-pointed punctum dilator or the point of a safety pin may locate the canaliculus. If it does not, use of a punctum dilator with not quite as sharp a point may succeed. If the punctum only is stenosed, the task of making an opening usually is not difficult.

A mildly stenosed punctum may respond to extremely gentle, repeated dilations. In most instances creating a permanent opening is simple, and the results are permanent. I prefer the technique using the Holth punch.

Acquired stenosis of canaliculus

Acquired stenosis of the canaliculus may have an acute onset, as in acute herpes simplex that involves the punctum and canaliculus, or a slow onset, as in trachoma. The stenosis may be partial, in which case fluid can be irrigated through the canaliculus into the nose, or it may be complete.

An "essential" type of stenosis that develops slowly over a period of months or years, primarily in middle life or later, is fairly common; most frequently, this begins in the region of the common canaliculus. Thickening of the subepithelial tissues in this area to cause a progressive narrowing of the lumen may be the major etiologic factor. The fact that the common canaliculus passes through the deep fascia to empty into the lacrimal sac may contribute to the narrowing. An entire canaliculus or all four may become completely stenosed.

Proper evaluation of the problem is not always easy. The dye test will usually be negative if the partial stenosis is sufficiently severe to cause epiphora. The Schirmer test is advisable to determine approximately the amount of tears secreted. If all of the irrigating fluid returns back through the punctum into which it is being instilled, the stenosis is in the canaliculus temporal to the common canaliculus. If all fluid irrigated into the lower canaliculus seems to return through the upper canaliculus, the obstruction is at the ampullary portion of the common canaliculus, or the patient has only a small obstructed lacrimal sac. The appearance of any shreds of mucus suggests that the problem is a small obstructed sac. Dacryocystography is indicated whenever there is any doubt.

Probably the most overlooked cause of epiphora is partial stenosis of the common canaliculus. The patient will taste the portion of the isotonic saline that flows into the nose when it is irrigated into the lower canaliculus. If the examiner or an assistant holds the upper lid upward to expose the upper punctum while irrigating fluid through the lower canaliculus, fluid will be seen exiting through the upper punctum. Only a few of these patients will have spontaneous fluorescein drainage that indicates they have at least some spontaneous tear drainage. The common canaliculus is functionally closed to tear drainage in most of these patients. The examiner is misled because fluid enters the nose under mild pressure. The importance of ascertaining if fluid injected through the lower canaliculus exits through the upper cannot be overemphasized.

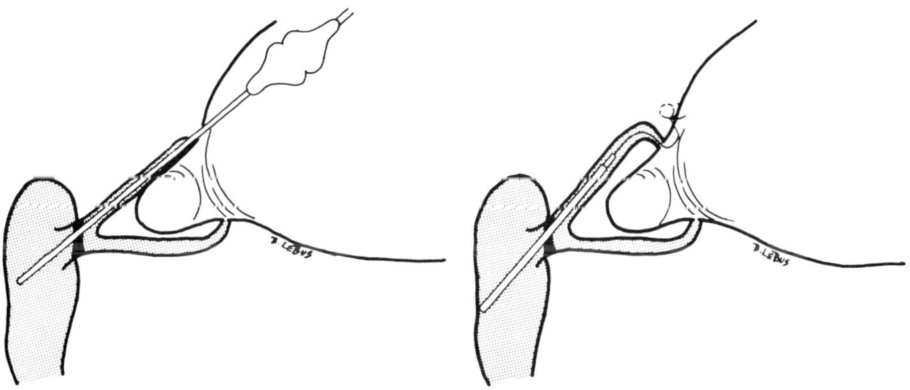

Fig. 5-14. Treatment of stenosis of ampullary portion of common canaliculus. *Left,* No. 1 Bowman probe is passed through stenosed ampullary portion of common canaliculus. *Right,* Stainless steel canalicular rod has been inserted. With needle threaded onto 4-0 silk exiting from upper punctum, bite is taken into soft tissues adjacent to punctum and knot is tied. (From Veirs, E. R.: Arch Ophthalmol **81**:569-570, 1969. Copyright 1969, American Medical Association.)

Treatment of stenosis of common canaliculus (use of canalicular rod). If the obstruction is not severe, treatment can be performed relatively easily in the office. In properly selected cases the percentage of permanent cures should approach 75% or more. If the obstruction requires considerable force to penetrate, the rate of good results decreases sharply.[3] Lidocaine is injected with a 30-gauge needle to block the nasociliary nerve (see Chapter 9), and this usually will give adequate anesthesia. It is important to guide the needle horizontally and posteriorly, beginning just superior to the medial palpebral tendon and infiltrating along the bony medial orbital wall for a distance of about 25 mm. A small amount of lidocaine can be injected through the skin in the region of the common canaliculus. If the procedure is performed on an outpatient, it is wise to advise the patient that diplopia may be experienced for an hour or so after injection of the nasociliary nerve. The medial rectus muscle is often affected simultaneously. Patching the involved eye for an hour or so until the diplopia wears off is advised.

A no. 1 or 2 Bowman probe is passed through the upper punctum and downward through the upper canaliculus as the lid is held up and outward with the other hand. After it penetrates the stenosis of the ampullary portion of the common canaliculus (Fig. 5-14, *left*), the probe is withdrawn. Isotonic saline is irrigated through both upper and lower canaliculi to test the patency. If fluid flows freely into the nose, a stainless steel canalicular rod* is inserted into the upper canaliculus. The distal end of the canalicular rod extends into the lacrimal sac through the stenosed area; only the 4-0 silk swaged in the punctal end of the rod exits from the upper punctum (Fig. 5-14, *right*). The 4-0 silk exiting from the punctum is threaded onto a curved needle, and a stitch is taken in the skin adjacent to the punctum and a knot is tied. Three months later, the knot is cut, the suture is grasped, and the canalicular rod is pulled out. Occasionally, the skin becomes irritated where the suture is knotted. Instead of anchoring the rod in position by suturing to the skin, the silk can be knotted into a ball too large to enter the punctum.

Another variation of anchoring the suture is to take a bite in the skin just superior to the punctum. The needle is continued upward subcutaneously for 6 to 8 mm before it is brought to the surface. A knot is then tied to anchor the suture in place. In other words, the knot will be just below the brow. If the knot becomes accidentally untied and the canalicular rod tends to slip downward too far into the sac, sufficient length of suture remains outside the punctum so that the canalicular rod can be easily pulled out.

Treatment of severe canalicular stenosis. If the amount of tear formation is minimal with resulting minimal epiphora, the patient probably should be encouraged to accept this annoyance. When the amount of epiphora causes a considerable irritation and becomes at least partially disabling, construction of an entirely new drainage channel is indicated (see Chapter 10).

*This is the same type of rod that is used for repair of freshly severed canaliculi (see Chapter 10).

REFERENCES

1. Jacobs, H. B.: Epiphora due to weak lid muscles, Br J Ophthalmol 43:332-339, 1959.
2. Kalt, E., and Kalt, M.: Cited by Duke-Elder, S.: Diseases of the lacrimal passages. In System of ophthalmology, vol. XIII, St. Louis, 1974, The C. V. Mosby Co., pp. 693-699.
3. Veirs, E. R.: Stenosis of the common canaliculus. Correction with a canalicular rod, Arch Ophthalmol 81:569-570, 1969.

CHAPTER 6

Etiology of dacryocystitis

With few exceptions, dacryocystitis is the result of obstruction in any part of the tear drainage system that extends from the upper part of the lacrimal sac to the lower end of the nasolacrimal duct. Except in the very young (in whom the cause is congenital occlusion, which usually opens spontaneously), dacryocystitis almost never resolves spontaneously. In rare cases an obstructing dacryolith may slide into the nose, relieving the obstruction.

CHRONIC DACRYOCYSTITIS

Chronic dacryocystitis is seen much more commonly than the acute form. The usual causes will be described.

Congenital occlusion of nasolacrimal duct

In this case, chronic low-grade dacryocystitis probably begins shortly after birth. Other than epiphora, the signs may be minimal.

Trauma

Midfacial fractures, especially from automobile accidents, that are not recognized and corrected may result in permanent obstruction within the sac. This trauma usually involves the nasoethmoid region at the level of the bony orbital margin (this is the junction of the lacrimal sac and nasolacrimal duct). Stranc[1] described obstruction in the nasolacrimal duct resulting from failure to recognize obstructions at this level that were due to fractures or that resulted from compression by inaccurately reduced bone fragments. Trauma from probing (except in the very young with congenital occlusion of the nasolacrimal duct) often converts a minimal nasolacrimal duct obstruction to a complete one with permanent dacryocystitis (until corrected surgically).

Dacryoliths

Dacryocystitis is always active when dacryoliths are present, and they occur in 10% to 20% of patients with dacryocystitis. Fungi can be cultured from many of the dacryoliths. Chemically, there are two groups of dacryoliths: (1) those that contain amino acids and are hydrophobic (cystine, lysine, histidine, glutamic acid, leucine, isoleucine, valine, phenylalanine, isoleucine) and (2) those that do not contain amino acids.

Dacryoliths may be discharged from the sac into the nose through the nasolacrimal duct, but this is uncommon. One of my patients discharged dacryoliths over a period of 10 years, remaining relatively free of symptoms for varying periods after each discharge. The fungi frequently cultured from the dacryoliths could be the etiologic factor in causing their formation. The nasolacrimal duct is nearly always patent, but the dacryoliths usually will re-form with recurrence of the dacryocystitis unless a large anastomosis is made from the lacrimal sac into the nose at the time the dacryoliths are removed.

Nasal and sinus disorders

Chronic infections, recurrent colds, nasal polyps, and sinusitis provide situations in which infection could readily travel upward through the nasolacrimal duct into the sac. Patients often mention symptoms suggestive of dacryocystitis during bouts of nasal or sinus infection, especially if they have had previous mild lacrimal involvements. These episodes of infection most likely cause a membranous closure of the nasolacrimal duct, which initially reopens after the infection subsides. There is, however, an increasing narrowing until a permanent cicatricial closure results. Chronic dacryocystitis follows.

Tumors and foreign bodies

These are infrequent causes of dacryocystitis, especially foreign bodies.

Idiopathic dacryocystitis

This is by far the most common type. These cases of chronic dacryocystitis have several interesting features: (1) most occur in women (male-to-female ratio, 1:8 to 1:9); (2) in most the onset is in middle age; and (3) many of these patients have greatly thickened, and at times markedly vascular, lining submucosa.

Bacteriologic considerations

The bacterial involvement plays second fiddle from a practical point of view, it seldom makes any difference which bacterium is causing the inflammation. The real problem is obstruction to the tear drainage, and treatment should be directed toward relieving that. I have seldom found antibiotics useful, before or after operation. Antibiotic therapy may be helpful in quieting down an acute infection. If surgical treatment is not to be performed, topical antibiotic drops and massage over the sac may keep the eye from being "messy."

ACUTE DACRYOCYSTITIS

Acute dacryocystitis may result from any of several causes, but all cases that I have seen have had one thing in common, namely, obstruction at the upper end of the lacrimal sac as well as at the lower end. The following etiologic factors seem to be the most common.

Chronic dacryocystitis

Acute dacryocystitis may be a sequela of the chronic form, usually of long (years) duration. Most of these patients have acquired idiopathic obstruction of the nasolacrimal duct (cicatricial closure of the duct). The chronic infection may persist for 20 or more years before the first acute attack occurs; recurrences at unpredictable intervals are the rule. During the acute attack the content of the lacrimal sac cannot be expressed by massage over the sac or fluid cannot be injected into the canaliculus because of temporary complete closure of the

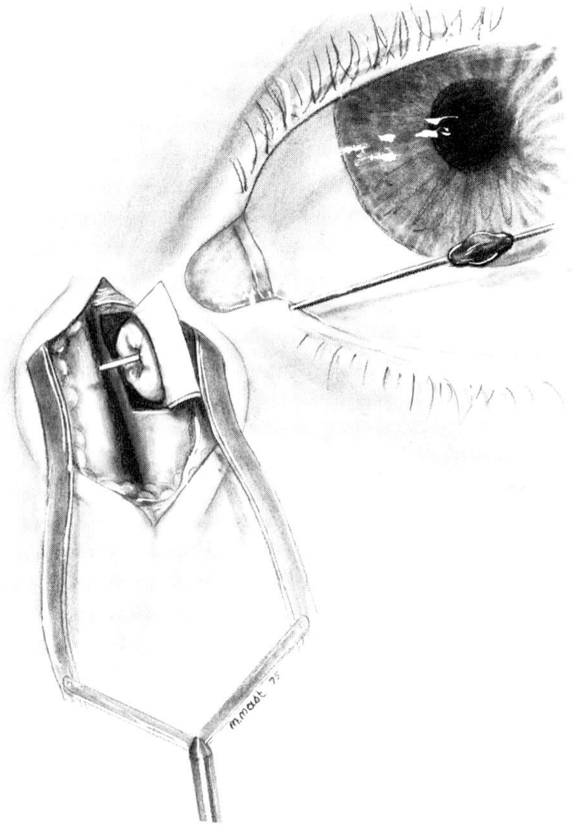

Fig. 6-1. Enlarged, edematous common punctum (where the common canaliculus empties into the lacrimal sac) is sometimes found at dacryocystorhinostomy. An increase in the inflammatory process would cause temporary complete closure. With permanently stenosed lacrimal duct, mucopus would have no way to escape, and an acute, painful swelling of the lacrimal sac would occur.

common canaliculus (sometimes a minimal amount can be injected in a few patients). However, the fluid contents of the sac can be withdrawn through the skin. A small amount of lidocaine is injected into the skin where it is most swollen. A 22-gauge needle attached to a 2-ml syringe is easily passed into the sac. After the sac fluid has been withdrawn, irrigation fluid can then be easily injected into the sac through the canaliculi. In many of these cases this is easily explained at later dacryocystorhinostomy: a small doughnutlike opening may be seen where the common punctum empties into the sac (Fig. 6-1).

Lacrimal sac valves or folds adjacent to common canaliculus opening

One of my patients had suffered from epiphora for more than 20 years but for about 1 year before operation had had repeated attacks of acute dacryocystitis. A large amount of pus could be expressed with some difficulty by massage over the sac. The dacryocystogram outlined only the superior portion of the lacrimal sac. A distinct large "valve" was found within the sac, obstructing the common canalicular opening.

Dacryoliths

To be responsible for the development of acute dacryocystitis, dacryoliths must obstruct the upper as well as the lower opening of the lacrimal sac. This

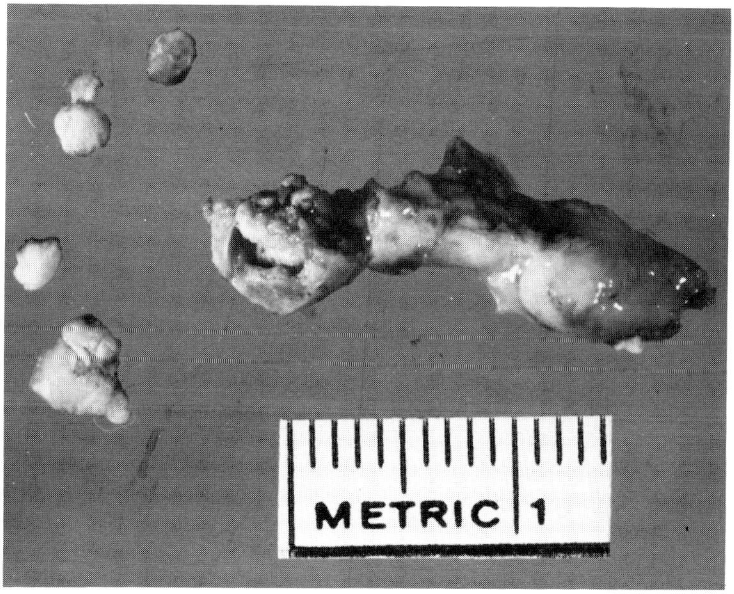

Fig. 6-2. Specimen from patient with long history of chronic dacryocystitis followed by intermittent attacks of acute dacryocystitis. Dacryolith extended from opening of common canaliculus into sac superiorly. Acute attacks occurred when dacryolith intermittently blocked common punctum superiorly.

may occur with a large single dacryolith that blocks the opening of the common canaliculus superiorly and the nasolacrimal duct inferiorly (Fig. 6-2). In other cases one dacryolith may lie in the lower portion of the lacrimal sac, effectively blocking the nasolacrimal duct, with another dacryolith in a "pocket" at the upper end of the sac blocking the opening of the common canaliculus. In one patient suffering from episodes of acute dacryocystitis, a valve or fold at the junction of the upper third and the lower two thirds of the sac divided the sac into two connecting compartments, each containing a dacryolith.

Trauma

Acute dacryocystitis that results from trauma may present a complicated picture, but as with other cases of acute dacryocystitis, obstruction occurs at both ends of the lacrimal sac. Usually, fracture of the facial bones has occurred, and most such patients give a history of one or more operative procedures. In one instance a 26-year-old woman who sustained facial injuries in a car wreck had undergone reconstructive surgery, which was followed by a chronic dacryocystitis. An attempt at dacryocystectomy failed (re-formation of the sac occurs in a high percentage of attempted dacryocystectomies, and except in instances of malignancies, removal of the sac is rarely indicated), and several severe attacks of acute dacryocystitis ensued. During an external dacryocystorhinostomy, the lacrimal sac was found to be enormously enlarged, especially laterally; the lower canaliculus was closed but the upper canaliculus was patent.

SUMMARY

Acute dacryocystitis seems to occur in patients who have chronic dacryocystitis due to an obstruction in the lower end of the sac and an obstruction (usually partial) in the upper end that blocks the escape of material from the sac through the canaliculi. Recurrence of the acute, and at times subacute, attacks is the rule until the predisposing condition is corrected surgically.

REFERENCE

1. Stranc, M. F.: The pattern of lacrimal injuries in naso-ethmoid fractures, Br J Plast Surg 23:339-346, 1970.

CHAPTER 7

Clinical manifestations of lacrimal sac disorders

Lacrimal sac disorders vary widely in their causes and character, and as might be expected, these disorders manifest themselves in a wide range of signs and symptoms. One feature that is common to most lacrimal disorders is that a cure rarely occurs spontaneously.

CHRONIC DACRYOCYSTITIS

Occurrence in infants and young children

Dacryocystitis secondary to congenital occlusion of the nasolacrimal duct usually manifests itself a few days after birth by epiphora and mucoid secretions within the conjunctival sac and by the eyelids being "matted" together on awakening. Rarely, the lacrimal sac will be enlarged at birth or soon after. Enlargement at birth probably is the result of accumulation of mucoid material in the sac prenatally. Infection within the sac occurs with time in all cases of congenitally occluded nasolacrimal duct. Rarely, an infant will develop an acute dacryocystitis with the signs of inflammation seen in adults with the condition.

The chronic infection of the sac seen in most infants who have an occluded nasolacrimal duct will maintain "messy" eyes with epiphora and mucoid secretions in the conjunctival sac and "matted eyelids" for weeks or months. The mucoid secretion or, more rarely, purulent material often can be expressed from the sac by massage over the sac. If the condition is unilateral, the appearance is much more striking. For a short time epiphora may be the only manifestation of an occluded duct in infants.

Spontaneous opening of the nasolacrimal duct occurs in many infants up to 3 or 4 months of age—almost the only time that spontaneous cure occurs when a lacrimal sac disorder is present. Symptoms disappear almost instantly after proper probing in infants under 6 to 12 months of age. Probing often is successful at an older age, up to 2 years or so.

Occurrence of unknown origin in adults (essential)

Age at onset. The vast majority of patients with dacryocystitis of unknown etiology will report onset at middle age or later. Dacryoliths will be found in a large percentage of patients who have onset of symptoms in the second or third decade of life and to a lesser extent in the fourth decade. One may question, and perhaps rightly, whether dacryocystitis associated with dacryoliths should be classified as sac involvement of unknown etiology—the dacryoliths being the cause of the dacryocystitis rather than just "the man who came to dinner." Dacryoliths are seen much more commonly in the age range when dacryocystitis is most prevalent, that is, middle age or older.

Signs and symptoms. Epiphora is always present. The amount depends on the amount of tears the patient would normally secrete were the lacrimal drainage system normal. A younger patient usually will have more severe epiphora than will an elderly one because the young secrete more tears, but there can be notable exceptions. For example, many elderly, weepy individuals may secrete an enormous amount of tears. Also, the severity of the sac infection may influence the amount of tear secretion: the more severe the infection, the more likely that reflex stimulation of tear secretion will increase the epiphora.

Mucopus or suppuration may be present with wide variations in degree. In the mildest form, sometimes called "silent dacryocystitis," the symptoms, including mucopus and epiphora, will be so minimal as to be hardly noticeable to the patient. Mucopus in the conjunctival sac and accompanying inflammation may not be evident to the examining physician. Usually, at least a minimal amount of mucopus can be lavaged from the sac. The bacteriostatic activity of the tears undoubtedly helps keep the infection to a minimum. However, most patients with chronic dacryocystitis will have symptoms almost constantly. Tears have to be wiped from the eyes every few minutes. Conjunctivitis is present, varying in degree from patient to patient and in the same patient at different times.

Symptoms will vary from time to time. An acute upper respiratory infection may cause an exacerbation of the sac infection. In some patients the symptoms may be minimized by routinely massaging over the lacrimal sac to cause the contents (mucopus or pus) to be regurgitated into the conjunctival sac, thus keeping the infection minor.

Oral or systemic administration of antibiotics is not indicated for chronically infected sacs unless complications develop. At best, the antibiotics bring only the infection under control as manifested by temporary disappearance of the conjunctivitis and by the expression of a clear viscous material rather than mucopus from the lacrimal sac. I have yet to see any advantage in administering antibiotics systemically prior to external dacryocystorhinostomy in patients with dacryocystitis. Removal of the cause, the obstruction to lacrimal drainage, results in a quick and uneventful cure.

Swelling of lacrimal sac region. An enlargement of the lacrimal sac sufficient to be palpated or seen grossly rarely occurs as a result of chronic dacryocystitis of unknown origin, regardless of its duration. The lacrimal fascia tightly attached to the anterior and posterior lacrimal crests is reinforced superiorly by the medial palpebral tendon and forms a strong barrier against expansion of the lacrimal sac outward beyond the lacrimal fossa. Tenderness on palpation over the lacrimal sac and pain may be encountered to a minimal degree with chronic essential dacryocystitis.

Occurrence secondary to recognizable pathologic processes

The many recognizable causes for chronic dacryocystitis are likely to produce various signs and symptoms. Neoplastic (benign and malignant) and nonneoplastic tumors, as in other types of dacryocystitis, have epiphora as a common denominator. Many tumors will produce swelling, usually irreducible, of the lacrimal sac below the medial palpebral tendon, and less often, above this tendon. Constant swelling of the sac above the tendon is almost pathognomonic of a lacrimal sac tumor. The amount of infection associated with sac tumors varies widely.

Midface injuries from blunt trauma occasionally will cause dacryocystitis as a result of bone fractures occluding the lower portion of the lacrimal sac or the nasolacrimal duct. The usual manifestations of essential dacryocystitis may be seen. Rarely, a draining lacrimal sac fistula through the skin may be one of the manifestations.

ACUTE DACRYOCYSTITIS

The clinical manifestations of acute dacryocystitis are much more dramatic in their onset and subsequent course than are those of chronic dacryocystitis.

The signs and symptoms of acute dacryocystitis will be better understood if the physician understands the pathologic processes responsible for the acute attacks. This was discussed more fully in Chapter 6. Simply stated, for the acute attack of dacryocystitis to occur, an obstruction must be present inferiorly (nasolacrimal duct or in the lower portion of the lacrimal sac) and superiorly (usually at the common punctum, where the canaliculus empties into the sac). The lower obstruction usually is a permanent cicatricial closure, whereas the upper obstruction usually is an incomplete closure that becomes functionally complete intermittently.

Age at onset. The first attack of acute dacryocystitis most often occurs in patients who have had chronic dacryocystitis for months or years, sometimes for 20 years or more. Because chronic dacryocystitis of the essential type occurs most often in middle-aged or older persons and is more frequent in women, acute dacryocystitis will be seen most often in these persons. However, acute dacryocystitis can occur at any age and is attributed to specific causes such as midfacial fractures or the presence of dacryoliths.

Signs and symptoms. The first symptom of an acute attack of dacryocystitis

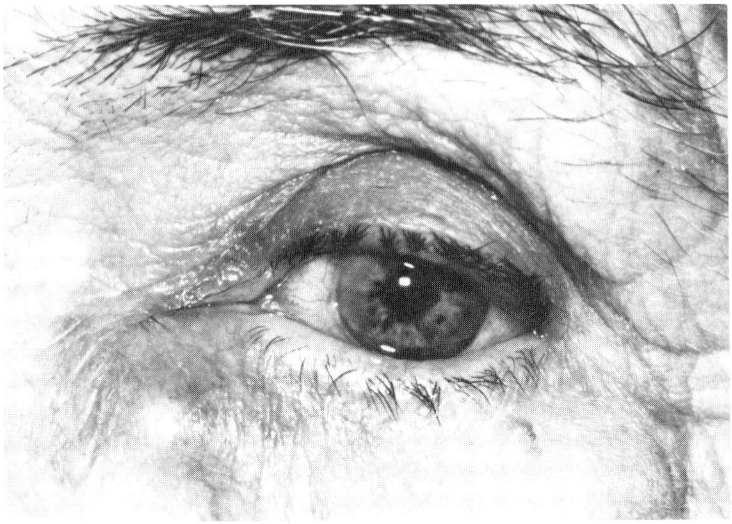

Fig. 7-1. Acute dacryocystitis. Swelling is maximal over lacrimal sac below medial palpebral tendon and also extends outward in all directions.

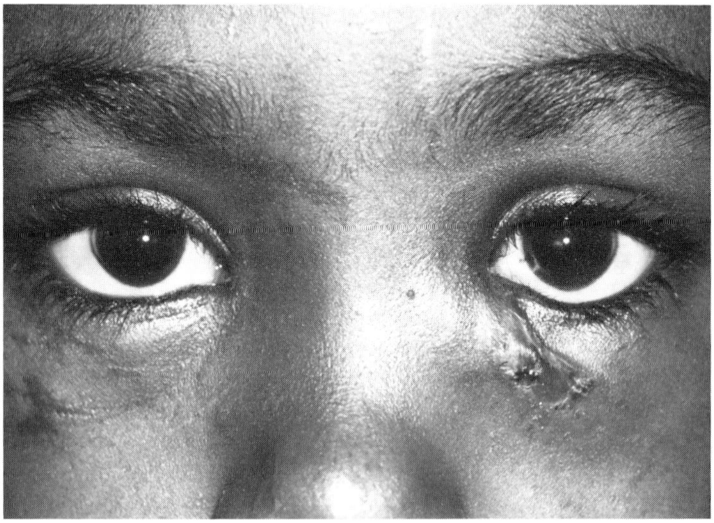

Fig. 7-2. Acute dacryocystitis with draining fistula.

is pain in and around the lacrimal sac, accompanied by tenderness. The pain may vary from mild to severe. The tenderness will also vary from mild to marked. Edema and injection of the sac area usually develop early. The swelling and redness may be mild or extend in all directions from the sac (Fig. 7-1). The patient will feel ill during a severe attack until resolution begins; milder attacks may cause only localized symptoms.

The reason for the acute pain is that the fascia that surrounds the sac is strong and tightly attached to the anterior and posterior lacrimal crests. In addition, on the superior aspect the medial palpebral tendon forms an impregnable barrier to any spontaneous expansion of the sac. The inflammatory contents of the sac are trapped within the sac and have no escape, causing increasing pain as the pressure builds up. Pressure over the sac will not cause the sac contents to regurgitate into the conjunctival sac because of the increased edema of the common canaliculus. In milder cases or as resolution develops, massage over the sac may result in some pus being regurgitated.

The tense, rigid sac may develop a spontaneous softness and fluctuation caused by the weakening of the fascia surrounding the sac. This can occur during the first acute attack of dacryocystitis or during subsequent attacks. In a few instances, there is a rupture from the sac through all the soft tissues inferior to the medial palpebral tendon, which results in a draining fistula through the skin (Fig. 7-2). Resolution of the acute attack occurs fairly rapidly with drainage.

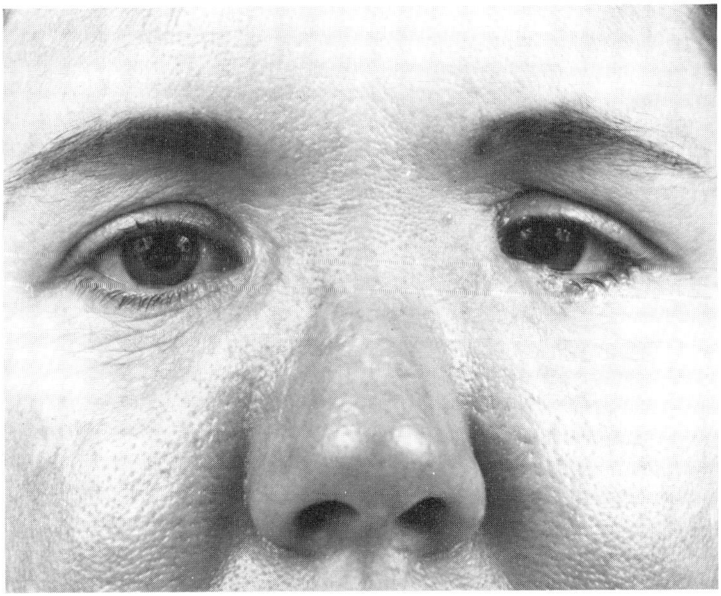

Fig. 7-3. Posttraumatic subacute dacryocystitis.

Occasionally, when the acute attack is severe and resolution is slow with treatment, a stab incision through the skin into the sac will give almost immediate relief. The pus can be withdrawn from the sac with a 23-gauge needle and syringe. After this, isotonic saline can be easily injected into the sac through the canaliculus. This demonstrates that the upper obstruction is relative. Dacryocystograms may be taken during an acute attack by using this technique, first drawing out the contents of the sac with a needle inserted directly into the sac through the skin and then injecting contrast medium into the sac through the canaliculus (see Chapter 8).

Attacks of acute dacryocystitis are more likely to be mild when the cause is the presence of dacryoliths obstructing the nasolacrimal duct and the common punctum or when it is a sequela of trauma (Fig. 7-3). The signs and symptoms in these cases are not so likely to be severe, but the course is likely to be more drawn out. Many of these cases should be classified as subacute dacryocystitis.

One important thing to remember is that with unusual exceptions, *once the patient has had an acute attack of dacryocystitis, acute attacks will continue to recur until there is adequate surgical intervention.*

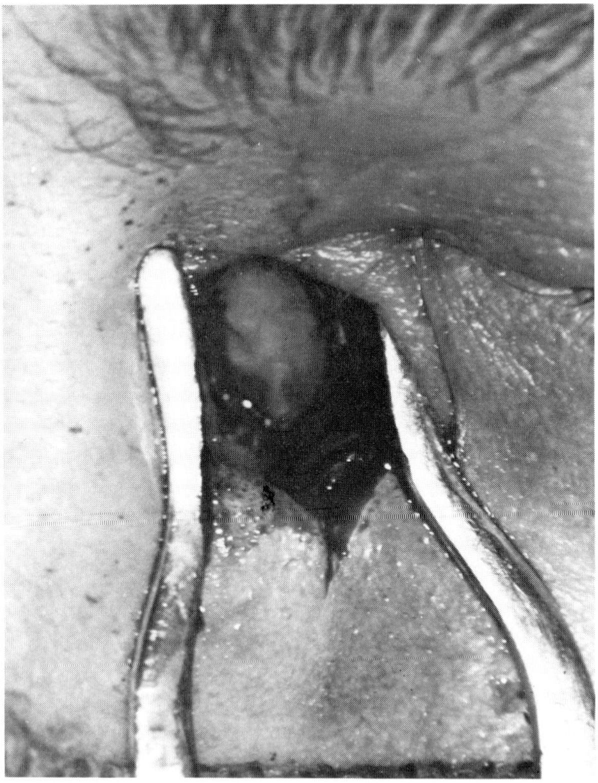

Fig. 7-4. Enormously enlarged mucocele completely occluding lacrimal sac. Epiphora disappeared after operation on mucocele.

TUMORS OF THE LACRIMAL SAC

Tumors, benign or malignant, involving the lacrimal sac are rare. Most originate within the lacrimal sac, and if benign, they usually will remain confined to the sac. Malignant tumors are likely to spread beyond the confines of the sac if not treated. Highly malignant tumors may involve not only the sac but also surrounding structures (sinuses, nose, and orbit) by the time the diagnosis is made. This usually makes the determination of their origin impossible. Conversely, tumors originating outside the lacrimal sac (from the nose, sinuses, or orbit) may enlarge sufficiently to involve the sac (Fig. 7-4).

Guerry and Smith[1] described three patients who presented with typical orbital mucoceles. Subsequent histopathologic studies revealed that in all three patients the paranasal sinus contained concomitant squamous cell carcinoma.

Tumors originating in adjacent skin, especially basal cell epithelioma, may destroy the lacrimal sac (Fig. 7-5).

Clinical manifestations. During the early symptomatic stages, most lacrimal sac tumors will manifest themselves in a remarkably similar fashion. Unilateral epiphora is nearly always the first symptom. In the early stages and often in later ones, fluid can be lavaged through the sac into the nose. This patency may last for months or years, probably longer with benign or low-grade malignant tumors. Inflammatory symptoms are usually minimal with neoplastic lacrimal sac tumors. With nonneoplastic tumors, there is likely to be mucopus that can be lavaged from the sac or that is present within the conjunctival sac and results in local irritation. Sacs containing polyps are especially likely to have more

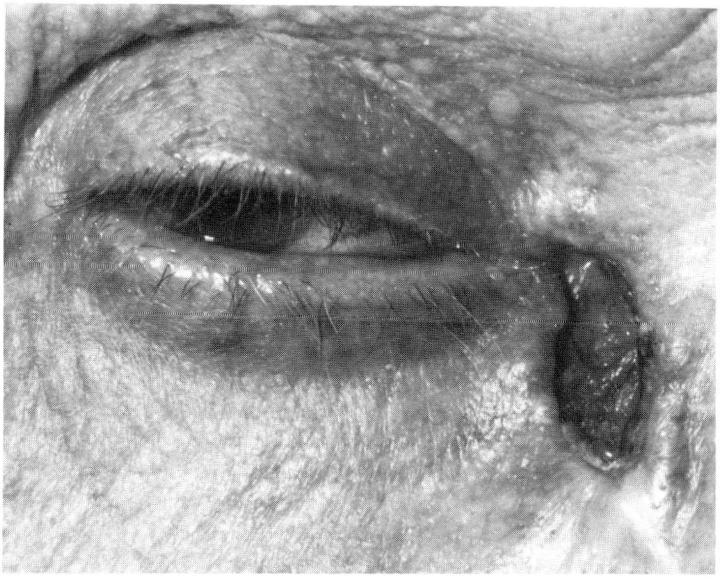

Fig. 7-5. Basal cell epithelioma, originating from skin, destroyed lacrimal sac.

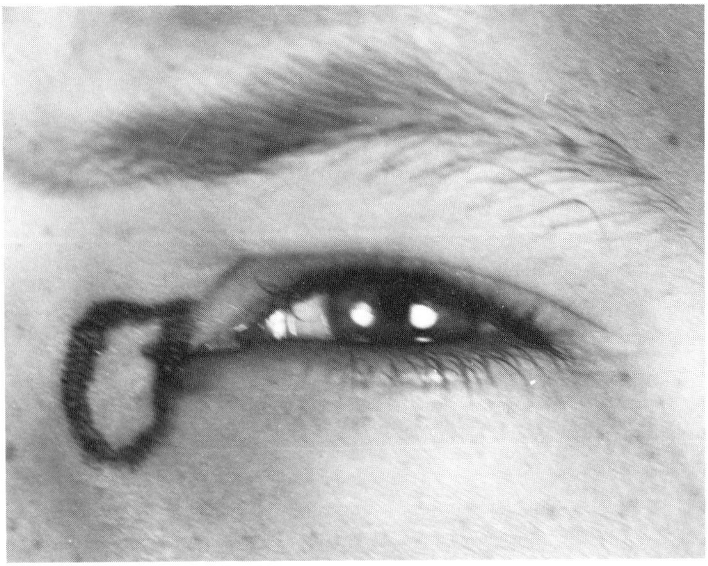

Fig. 7-6. Slowly developing tumor that could be palpated to extent outlined, which reached several millimeters superior to medial palpebral tendon. Patient had constant epiphora. Saline could be injected into nose only by occluding upper punctum and injecting through lower canaliculus under considerable pressure.

pronounced inflammatory symptoms; in these cases the nose often contains polyps, and the patients have a nasal allergy. Pain is not associated with sac tumors except with malignant neoplasms, and even then pain is not common.

A palpable, painless mass develops with varying degrees of rapidity when a lacrimal sac tumor develops. The mass occasionally is reducible by massage but only to a minimal extent. The induration detected by palpation is due not only to the tumor but also to the tautness of the deep facia that surrounds the sac, the fascia being securely attached to the anterior and posterior lacrimal crests. Most lacrimal sacs involved by acute infection also will feel indurated and are irreducible with massage because the sac contents cannot escape. Pain, tenderness on pressure, redness, and relatively short duration of symptoms suggest acute dacryocystitis rather than lacrimal sac tumor.

Extension of an irreducible lacrimal sac swelling to above the medial palpebral tendon is all but pathognomonic of a tumor involving the lacrimal sac (Fig. 7-6). Many lacrimal tumors do not cause swelling above the palpebral tendon (Fig. 7-7). Edema accompanying acute dacryocystitis may extend above the medial palpebral tendon but is easily recognizable and is inflammatory. Rarely, neoplastic tumors originating within the lacrimal sac will send a tongue of tumor migrating through a canaliculus, and it can be seen exiting at the punctum (Fig. 7-8). Fungi may cause a lacrimal sac tumor, although far more often fungi found in the sac are associated with dacryoliths and other "foreign" material.

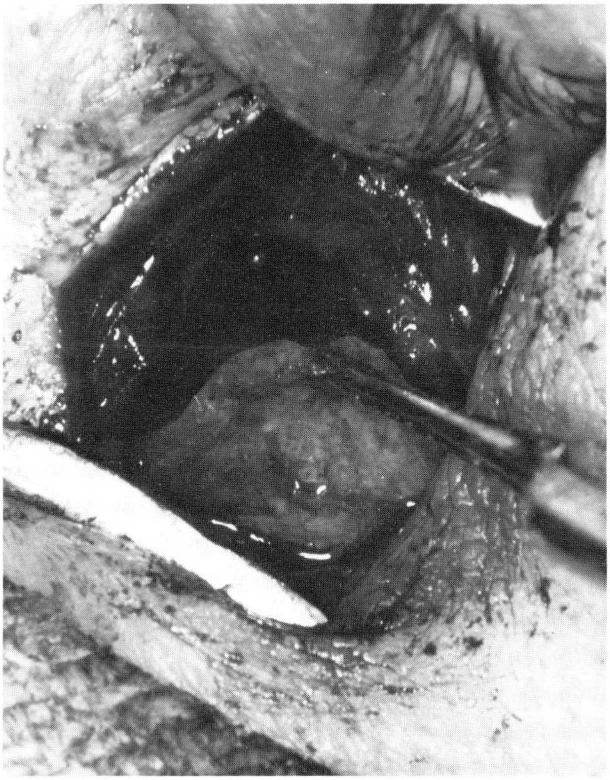

Fig. 7-7. Large granuloma, tightly bound to all of lacrimal sac lining, could be palpated only inferiorly to medial palpebral tendon. Epiphora and bleeding were the only symptoms. Part of tumor dissected loose is held by hook.

The vast majority of patients with sac tumors will have symptoms of varying degrees of severity when first seen. The duration of these symptoms varies from a few months to 20 years or more. The age range of these patients is wide. Approximately half of the tumors of the lacrimal sac are epithelial. A rare type of epithelial tumor is the mucoepidermoid carcinoma (Fig. 7-9). In a study of 27 patients with primary epithelial tumors of the lacrimal sac, Ryan and Font[2] found the median age to be 55 years; the age range was 9 to 89 years among patients with papillomas and 40 to 75 years among those with carcinomas.

Dacryocystography (see Chapter 8) may be helpful in a few cases by suggesting the presence of lacrimal sac tumors. More important, however, dacryocystography will demonstrate that some type of pathologic process exists that should be explored.

Diagnosis. The most reliable preoperative diagnostic sign of lacrimal sac tumors is a noninflammatory, irreducible swelling of the lacrimal sac that extends above the medial palpebral tendon, usually of long duration. However, most sac tumors do not extend above this tendon. Epiphora is always present but occurs

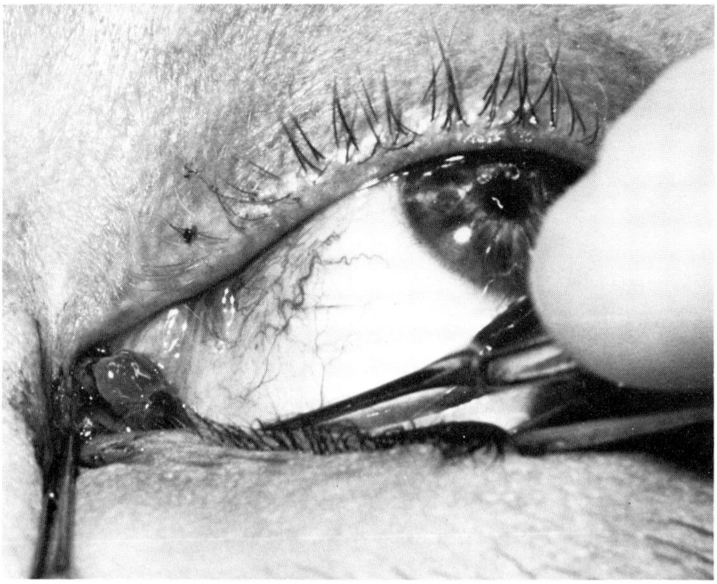

Fig. 7-8. Small tumor spontaneously extruding through upper punctum was repeatedly snipped off at punctum. Hemangioma shows through slit canaliculus. When lacrimal sac was opened, tumor filled sac and had small pediclelike attachment to sac wall near opening of common punctum. Removal of tumor was easy. Cautery was applied to area of origin. There were no recurrences.

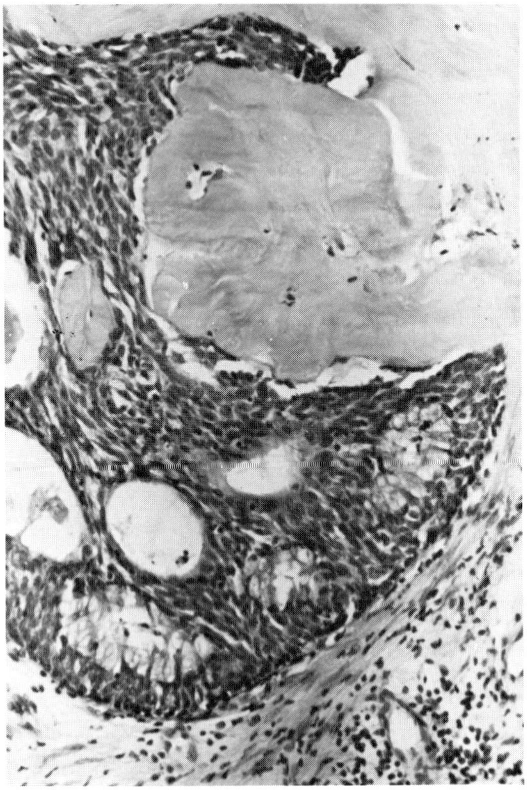

Fig. 7-9. Mucoepidermoid carcinoma of lacrimal sac, showing mixture of squamous epithelial cells associated with inspissated mucus. (Courtesy J. R. McFarlane, Jr., M.D., San Antonio, Texas.) (Hematoxylin and eosin, ×450.)

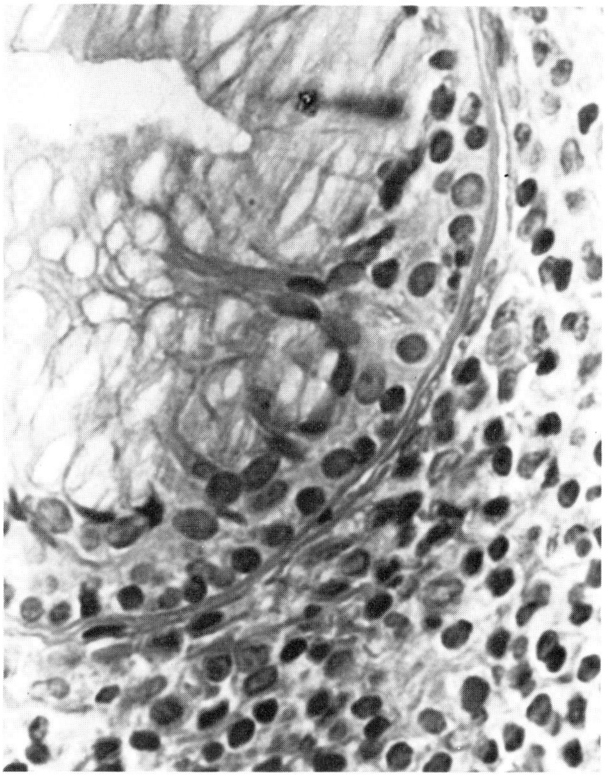

Fig. 7-10. Tumor of lacrimal sac. Gland is surrounded by neoplastic lymphocytes in patient with well-differentiated lymphocytic lymphoma. (Hematoxylin and eosin; ×800.)

commonly from many causes. Hemorrhages may occur. Dacryocystograms may show findings suggestive of tumors and should always be made when any pathologic process is suspected.

Treatment. Treatment of lacrimal sac tumors will depend on the type of tumor—whether intrinsic or extrinsic, whether benign or malignant—and on its size and location. Rarely is the diagnosis made until the lacrimal sac is opened. If lymphocytic lymphoma is diagnosed (Fig. 7-10), localized irradiation is given cautiously in addition to chemotherapy if indicated, especially if the patient has sufficient lacrimal symptoms to justify the treatment. Usually lymphoma of the sac is just one manifestation of a generalized disease.

Granulomas and other benign tumors may be tightly adherent to the sac wall. Careful dissection to avoid undue damage to other structures is used to remove as much of the tumor as possible. If fluid can be injected into the sac, an anastomosis can be made into the nose if there is any doubt about the future patency of the nasolacrimal duct. Leaving a specially constructed Pyrex tube in the anastomosis may be indicated (see Chapter 9). Some benign tumors may have a small pedicle whose base can be cauterized after the tumor is removed.

Removal of small, low-grade malignant tumors has to be individualized. If the patient is elderly or in poor health, excision of the tumor and thorough cauterization of the base may be the best course. If the tumor is more extensive, and especially if it has spread beyond the sac, more radical surgery is indicated. The more malignant tumors may spread extensively beyond the lacrimal sac, to the nose, paranasal sinuses, eyelids, and orbit. Extensive, mutilating surgery followed by radiation therapy may be tried. The prognosis is usually grave. With some rapidly growing sac malignancies, invasion of tissues may be so extensive that palliative irradiation may be the most humane treatment.

REFERENCES

1. Guerry, R. K., and Smith, J. L.: Paranasal sinus carcinoma causing orbital mucocele, Am J Ophthalmol 80:943-946, 1975.
2. Ryan, S. J., and Font, R. L.: Primary epithelial neoplasms of the lacrimal sac, Am J Ophthalmol 76:73-88, 1973.

CHAPTER 8

Dacryocystography

Dacryocystography is a simple, safe, and quick method by which one can obtain valuable information concerning the status of the lacrimal drainage system. It should be considered as an adjunctive diagnostic procedure to supplement information obtained by a thorough clinical examination of the patient's lacrimal system, including inspection of the puncta and conjunctiva, the use of the Schirmer and dye tests, massage over the lacrimal sac region, irrigation, and examination of the nose.

The dacryocystogram made preoperatively should be on the view box in the operating room at the time of operation. This will permit instant review, which could be helpful in performing the operation. In addition, a glance at the dacryocystogram prevents the unfortunate error of operating on the wrong side.

TECHNIQUE

The procedure usually is simple and should cause only minimal discomfort to the patient.

After the lacrimal sac has been emptied of as much of its contents as possible by massage over the sac, it is thoroughly irrigated with isotonic saline to remove residual mucoid or other material. The sac again is thoroughly emptied of its contents by massage before the radiopaque material is injected into it. This prevents globulation (Fig. 8-1), a condition caused by the fact that watery and oily solutions do not mix. For the most satisfactory result, injection of the contrast medium should be performed in the room where the roentgenograms are to be taken so that they can be made without unnecessary delay.

During acute attacks of dacryocystitis, frequently none of the sac content can be massaged from the sac, nor can any solution be injected into the sac through the canaliculi. During subacute attacks often only a small amount, if any, of the sac content can be expressed. This is because the common canalicular opening into the sac is obstructed as a result of edema, an obstructing "valve," or a dacryolith. A 25-gauge needle that is attached to a 2-ml syringe can easily be passed directly into the enlarged sac through the skin, and the contents of the sac can then be withdrawn. The contrast material can then be injected into the sac through the canaliculus (Fig. 8-2). This technique not only allows a good

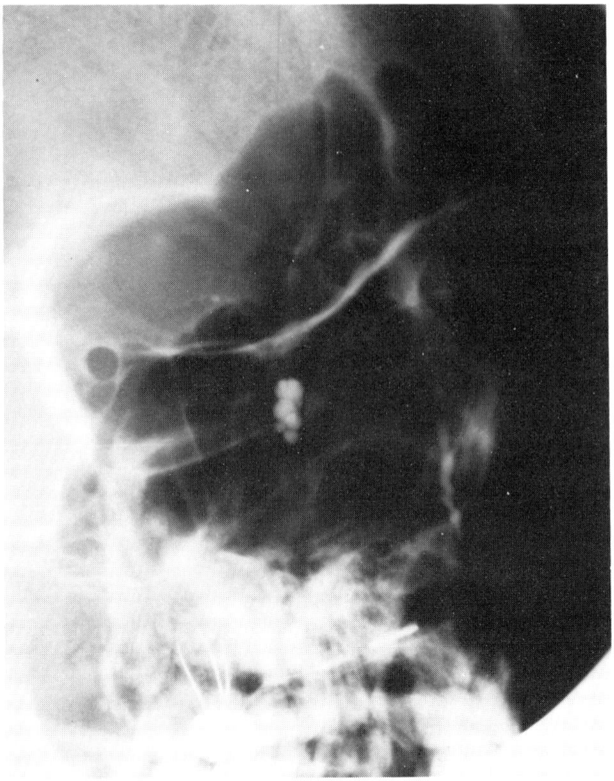

Fig. 8-1. Marked globulations on one side only in oblique view.

dacryocystogram to be taken but also indicates that tear drainage through the common canaliculus is likely to be adequate after an external dacryocystorhinostomy.

Iophendylate (Pantopaque) is a satisfactory contrast medium. It comes in a sterile 3-ml glass vial that provides an ample amount for injection bilaterally.

One or two drops of a topical anesthetic agent are placed in the conjunctival sacs, and the lower puncta are gently dilated with a punctal dilator. The contrast medium is injected from a 2-ml syringe fitted with a lacrimal tip through the lower canaliculus (the upper may be used if the lower is obstructed). The obstructed side is injected first because the contrast medium cannot readily escape from it. The other side is then injected. The patient can readily taste the contrast medium that flows through the lacrimal drainage system into the nose. The excess contrast material that collects in the inner canthal region is gently wiped away with a cotton-tipped applicator, and the patient is told not to rub his eyes.

The roentgenograms should be taken as soon as possible after the injection of the contrast material. Usually, the posteroanterior (Caldwell's) and oblique views are taken (Fig. 8-3). However, when the patient is an infant under general

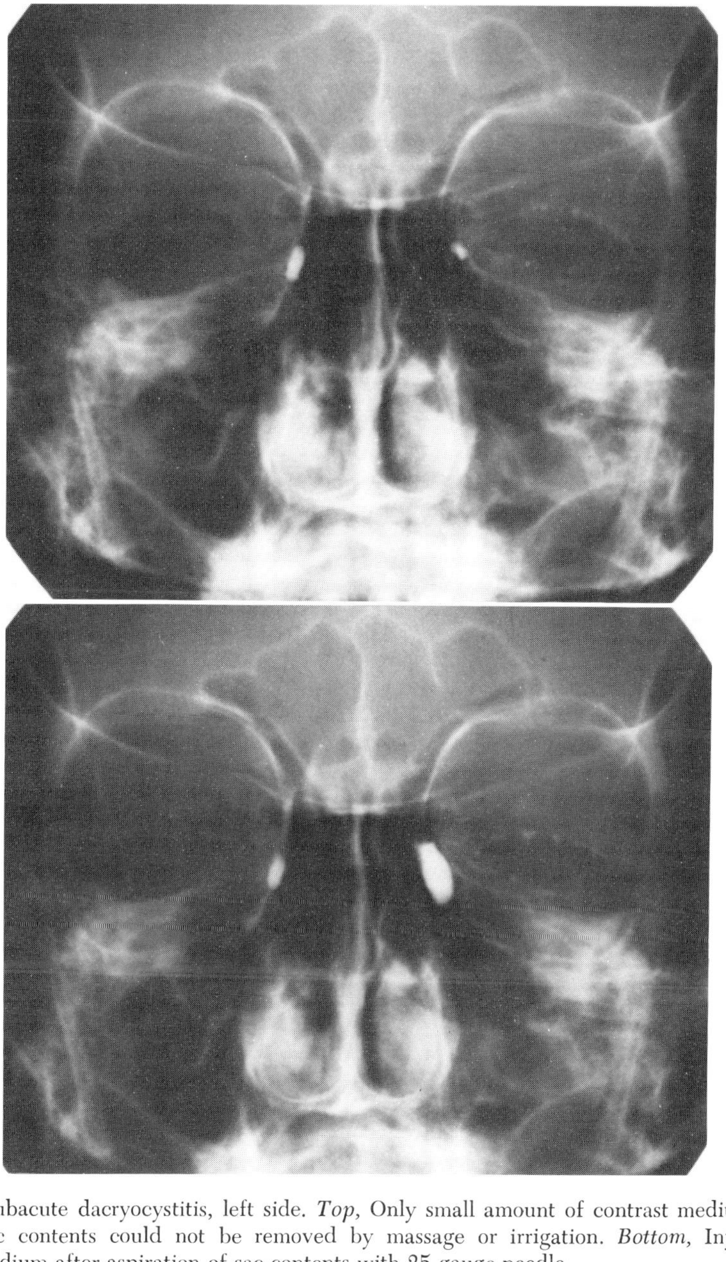

Fig. 8-2. Subacute dacryocystitis, left side. *Top,* Only small amount of contrast medium in sac because sac contents could not be removed by massage or irrigation. *Bottom,* Injection of contrast medium after aspiration of sac contents with 25-gauge needle.

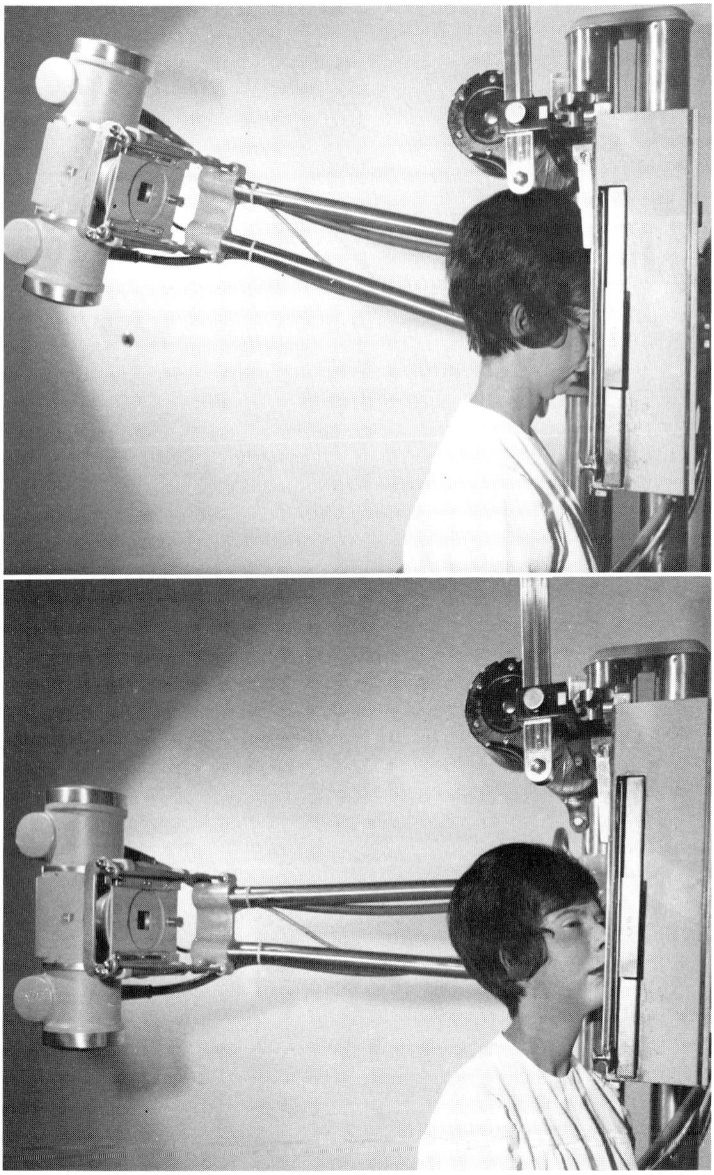

Fig. 8-3. Recommended roentgenographic views after injection of contrast medium. *Top,* Posteroanterior (Caldwell's) view. *Bottom,* Oblique view (optic canal view).

anesthesia, only an anteroposterior view may be practical. Because radiology technicians usually are familiar with taking the optic canal view, this is a satisfactory way to obtain an excellent oblique view. Only one optic canal view (right or left) is needed to show both ducts. Lateral views are unsatisfactory because the outlines of the two sides are superimposed.

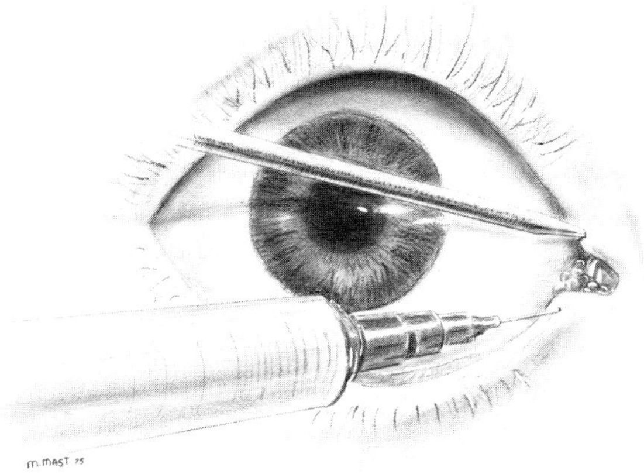

Fig. 8-4. Upper punctum is occluded during injection through lower punctum under mild pressure.

In some patients, such as those having a partial common canalicular stenosis or whose lacrimal sac contains a dacryolith or tumor, saline injected into the canaliculus may pass through the sac and enter the nose. A more viscous solution such as Pantopaque may enter the lacrimal sac unsatisfactorily or not at all when injected in this manner. Occluding the upper punctum with a punctal dilator while injecting the Pantopaque through the lower canaliculus under mild pressure will often produce satisfactory dacryocystograms (Fig. 8-4).

Cases that require injection under mild pressure are often the ones in which the dacryocystograms yield the most valuable information. Injection of the contrast material into the soft tissues may occur, especially if undue trauma causes penetration of the lacrimal ducts. But I have never been aware of this happening in many hundreds of dacryocystograms taken. Repeat roentgenograms may be taken 15 to 30 minutes after the injection of the contrast medium if determination of the emptying time is deemed important.

Intubation macrodacryocystography has been described by Lloyd and coworkers[2] and others. The lower canaliculus is usually catheterized for a distance of 3 to 4 mm, which allows continuous injection of the lacrimal drainage system as the roentgenograms are taken. Geometric enlargement of the roentgenographic image is obtained by placing the x-ray film some distance from the head. This technique has been recommended because it supposedly gives better demonstration of the lacrimal drainage system, especially for demonstrating lesions of the canaliculi preoperatively.

Putterman[3] described inserting a ⅝-inch 25-gauge needle inferiorly to the medial canthal tendon and posteriorly to the anterior lacrimal fossa. Through this, 0.5 ml of water-soluble contrast material such as Renografin is injected. If there is no swelling of the eyelids, an additional 1 ml is injected and a posteroanterior roentgenogram is quickly taken. No complications occurred because

Renografin is well tolerated and is rapidly absorbed if it extravasates into the tissues.

INTERPRETATION

Normal dacryocystogram

The normal lacrimal sac and nasolacrimal duct can be followed as a continuous "tube" of small diameter extending from the medial canthal tendon superiorly to its opening into the nose inferiorly. The sac and nasolacrimal duct slope posteriorly and laterally as they pass inferiorly. The diameter of the tube may increase as it passes inferiorly, with the maximal diameter beginning at the juncture of the lacrimal sac and the nasolacrimal duct. The lacrimal sac, which lies within the orbit, is approximately 2 cm in length, but the dacryocystogram demonstrates only that portion extending from the medial canthal tendon to the lacrimal sac–nasolacrimal duct junction.

As it passes inferiorly, the nasolacrimal duct is enclosed in bone for approximately 1 cm and then is surrounded by soft tissue for varying lengths until the duct empties into the nose under the inferior turbinate. The normal lacrimal sac is more of a potential space than a "tube" with a relatively uniform diameter. Instillation of an oily contrast medium enlarges the lacrimal sac slightly (Fig. 8-5). Many normal sacs will show a fairly uniform diameter, whereas others will show irregularities. The contrast material can be easily visualized in the nose. If he routinely takes bilateral dacryocystograms in every case of suspected

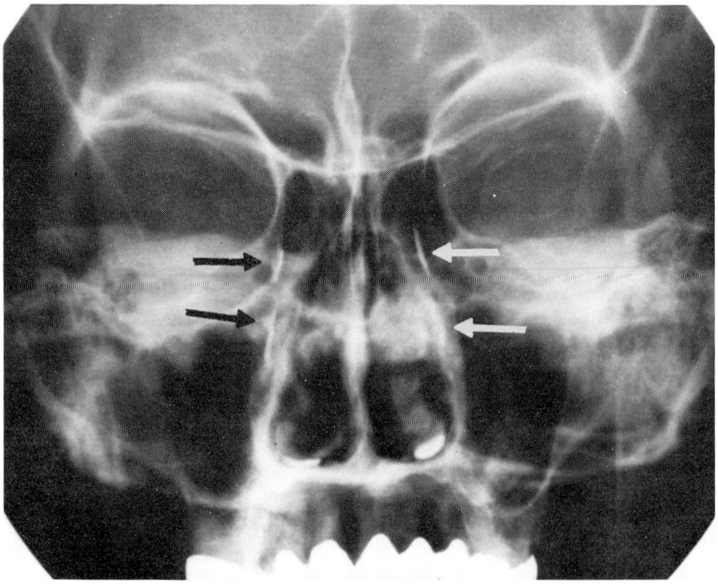

Fig. 8-5. Normal dacryocystogram, posteroanterior (Caldwell's) view.

lacrimal sac disorders, the ophthalmologist quickly learns to recognize a normal dacryocystogram.

Abnormal dacryocystogram

The history and physical findings are often helpful in the interpretation of abnormal dacryocystograms. If the signs and symptoms date from birth, congenital abnormalities should be suspected. If they follow trauma, the clinician should look carefully for evidence of old fractures of the midfacial bones.

Congenital abnormalities. Dacryocystograms are seldom indicated in infants with congenital occlusion of the nasolacrimal ducts because the majority can be cured by proper probing of the nasolacrimal ducts. In a few cases in infants less than 12 months old the condition will not respond to probing. Contrast material instilled into both sides while the infant is under general anesthesia often will reveal a greatly enlarged lacrimal sac with smooth outline (Fig. 8-6).

Dacryocystograms may be helpful in determining the degree of patency of the nasolacrimal duct before or after probing. Congenital fistulas are easily demonstrated.

Obstruction of canaliculus–lacrimal sac junction. When the contrast medium injected into the lower punctum exits instantly through the upper punctum, the obstruction is usually at the junction of the common canaliculus and the lacrimal sac. The outline of the canaliculi usually can be readily identified (Fig. 8-7).

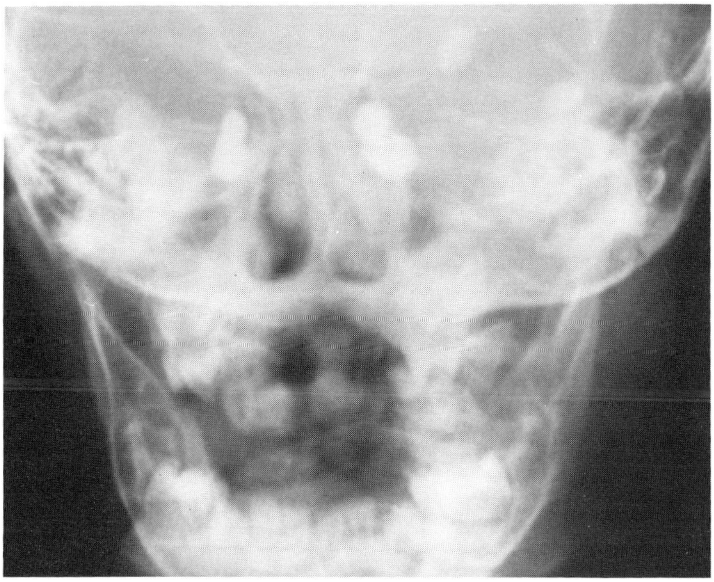

Fig. 8-6. Enlarged, totally obstructed lacrimal sacs in 6-month-old infant (roentgenogram taken while patient was on operating table under general anesthesia). Lacrimal ducts could not be probed. Possibility of congenital osseous occlusion rather than membranous occlusion.

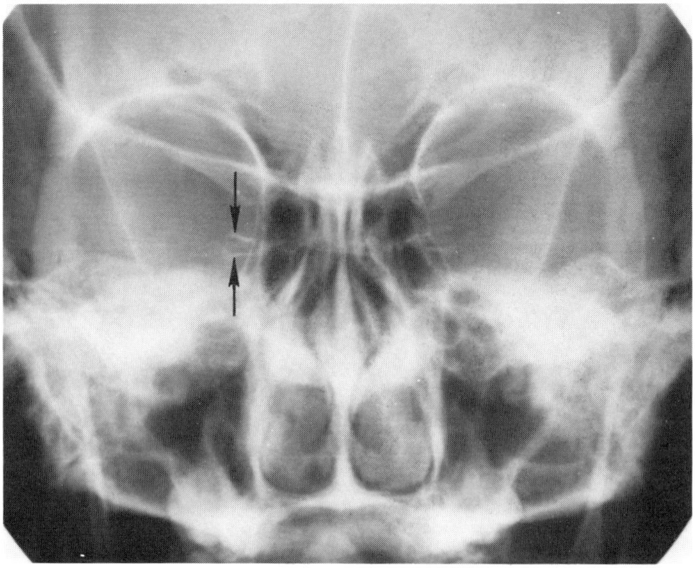

Fig. 8-7. Stenosis at junction of common canaliculus and lacrimal sac. Arrows point to outlines of canaliculi.

One of the most important uses of dacryocystography is to distinguish between obstruction at the canalicular-sac level and high-level lacrimal sac obstruction. With a high-level lacrimal sac obstruction, isotonic saline injected into the lower canaliculus will seem to exit instantly through the upper punctum, as will injected contrast medium; usually, only a small lacrimal sac is present. If even the smallest amount of mucoid material is lavaged out, this is strong evidence that the obstruction is within the sac. A dacryocystogram will confirm the diagnosis.

This differential diagnosis is exceedingly important. If even a small lacrimal sac is present, external dacryocystorhinostomy is likely to be successful. Stenosis involving the canaliculi requires a different technique for relief.

Size and level of lacrimal sac or nasolacrimal obstructions. The blockage may be at the lower end of the bony nasolacrimal duct (Fig. 8-8, *A*). Obstructions at the lower end of the lacrimal sac are not uncommon (Fig. 8-8, *B*).

The lacrimal sac may enlarge laterally, especially if the dacryocystitis is of long duration. Many sacs that have had repeated acute or subcute attacks of the infection frequently will become quite enlarged (Fig. 8-8, *C*).

Demonstration of a small lacrimal sac is a warning to the surgeon that fashioning a permanent functioning anastomosis is likely to be more difficult than with large sacs.

Determination of lacrimal sac configuration. Distinct multiple valves that can be demonstrated by dacryocystograms and confirmed at operation are rare

A

B

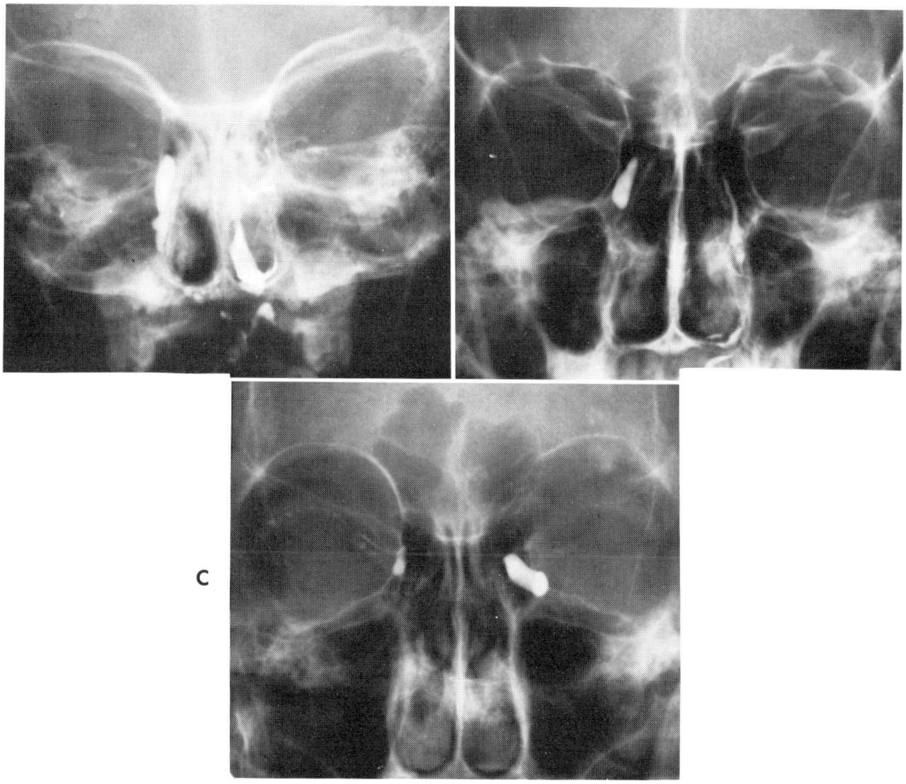

C

Fig. 8-8. Obstructions demonstrated by dacryocystography. **A,** Obstruction at lower end of nasolacrimal duct (congenital occlusion in 2-year-old child). **B,** Obstruction superior to lacrimal sac–nasolacrimal duct junction on patient's right side (patent duct on left side shows normal increase in diameter at junction). **C,** Marked lateral enlargement of lacrimal sac (84-year-old patient with history of repeated attacks of acute dacryocystitis).

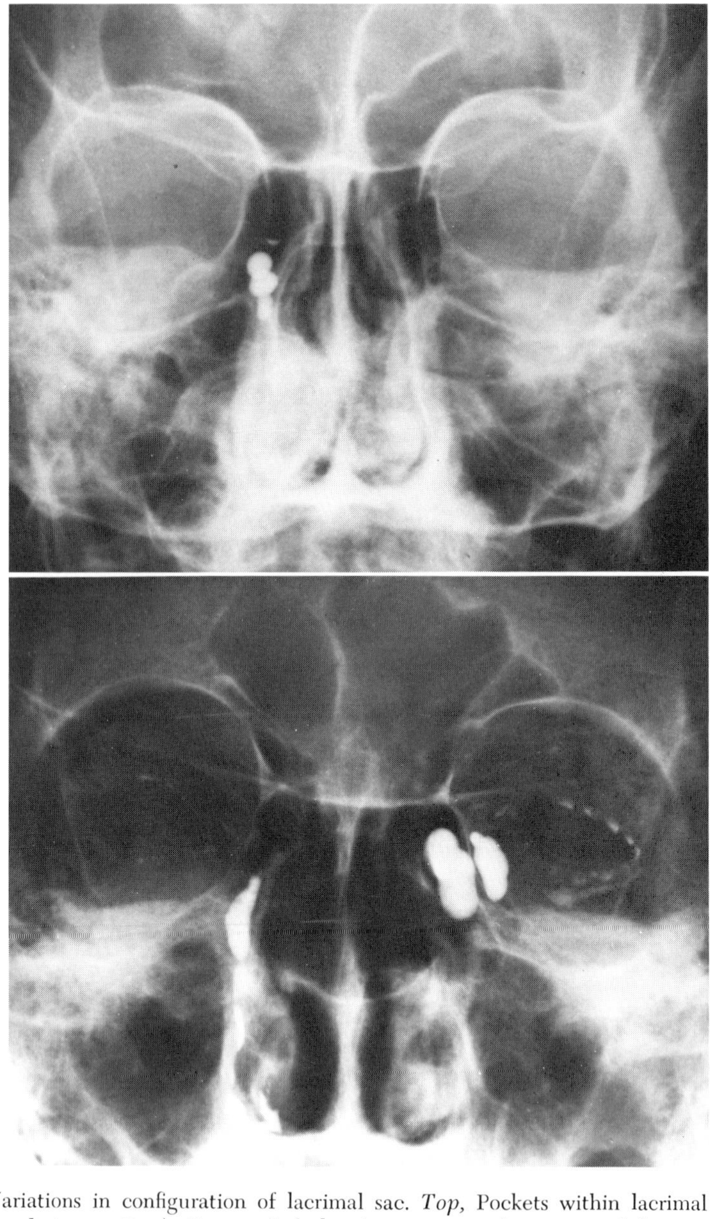

Fig. 8-9. Variations in configuration of lacrimal sac. *Top,* Pockets within lacrimal sac due to valves (proved at operation). *Bottom,* Lobulated appearance due to partial division of lacrimal sac in vertical direction by "septum." This septum was only about 2 mm high.

(Fig. 8-9, *top*). These should not be confused with globulations as shown in Fig. 8-1. Sometimes the dacryocystogram suggests that the lacrimal sac is divided into two separate parts by a vertical septum (Fig. 8-9, *bottom*).

DACRYOCYSTITIS AFTER TRAUMA

Midfacial trauma is not an infrequent cause of blockage of the lacrimal drainage system, and dacryocystitis is the aftermath of this obstruction. The obstruction most frequently is at the junction of the lacrimal sac and the nasolacrimal duct, but it may occur at any level. Blunt trauma, especially as a result of an automobile accident, causes fractures of the nasoethmoid region. Closure of the lacrimal drainage system frequently is not repaired soon after the injury because it goes unrecognized.

Gerlock[1] has reported that a roentgenogram taken in the axial projection will readily show the bony lacrimal canal (Fig. 8-10). In his technique the patient lies on the roentgenographic examining table in the supine position so that his head is in a submental vertex position and the canthomeatal line is parallel to the top of the table. A single exposure is made with the tube angled 12° cranially and the central ray centered over the inner margin of the symphysis menti.

If irrigation with isotonic saline indicates a blocked lacrimal passage, dacryocystograms made prior to the primary repair may be helpful. Because of the

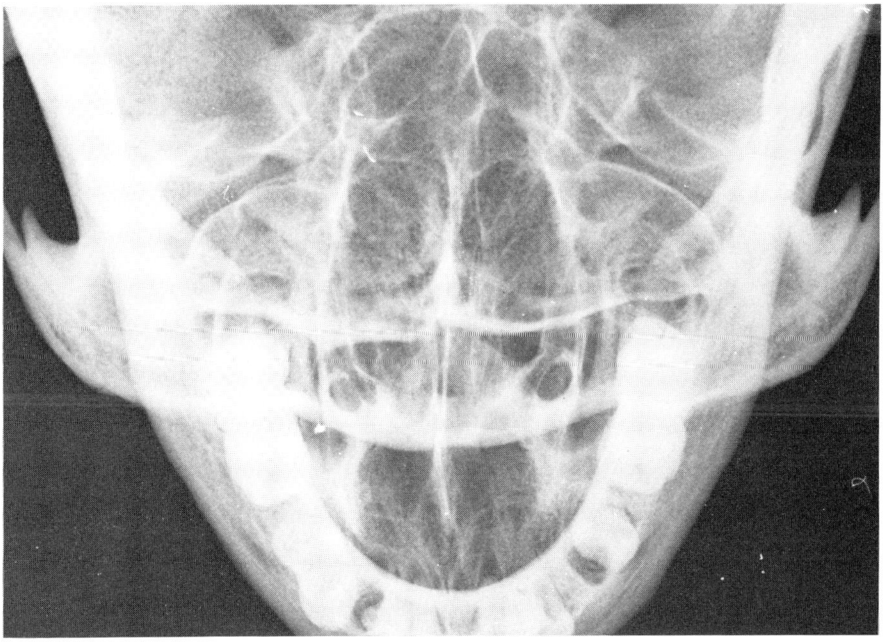

Fig. 8-10. Foramenlike appearance of bony lacrimal canals when viewed in axial projection. (From Gerlock, A. J., Jr.: South Med J 68:118-120, 1975.)

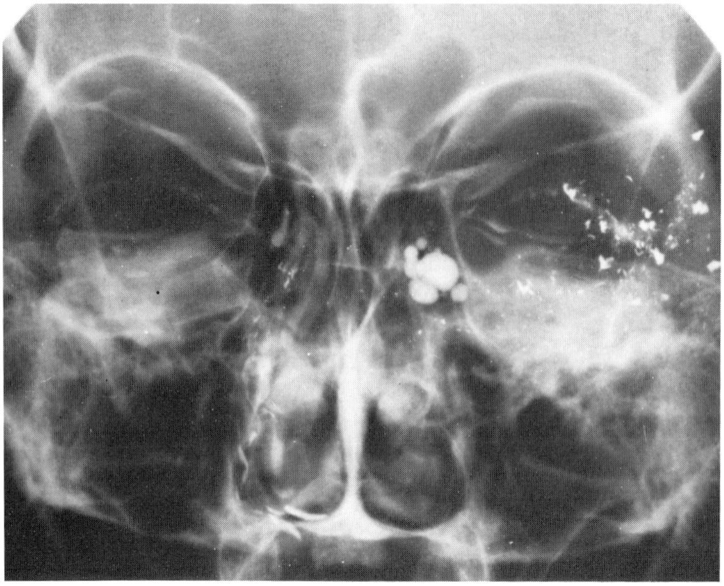

Fig. 8-11. Chronic dacryocystitis as sequela to gunshot wound. Globulations are result of incomplete removal of fluid before injection of contrast medium.

possibility of infiltrating the soft tissues with contrast medium soon after the injury, the injection should be done carefully. Unfortunately, the possibility of injury involving the lacrimal sac is seldom thought of at the time of the primary repair.

Gunshot wounds (Fig. 8-11), intranasal operations (most often to make a nasoantral window), and a wide variety of other injuries may result in dacryocystitis.

Dacryocystography may demonstrate a fistula extending from the lacrimal sac–nasolacrimal duct junction into the maxillary antrum. If the fistular connection is narrow, dacryocystitis may ensue (Fig. 8-12, *top*). If it is larger (Fig. 8-12, *bottom*), drainage into the maxillary antrum is adequate and dacryocystitis does not occur.

DACRYOLITHS

The presence of dacryoliths often can be suspected from the appearance of a dacryocystogram. More important than trying to determine the presence or absence of dacryoliths is the demonstration that some pathologic process does exist within the lacrimal sac. Because isotonic saline usually can be lavaged through the lacrimal drainage system even when dacryoliths are present, the conclusion is often drawn that no sac problem exists—despite symptoms of dacryocystitis.

Irregularity in the outline of a dilated lacrimal sac is most suggestive evi-

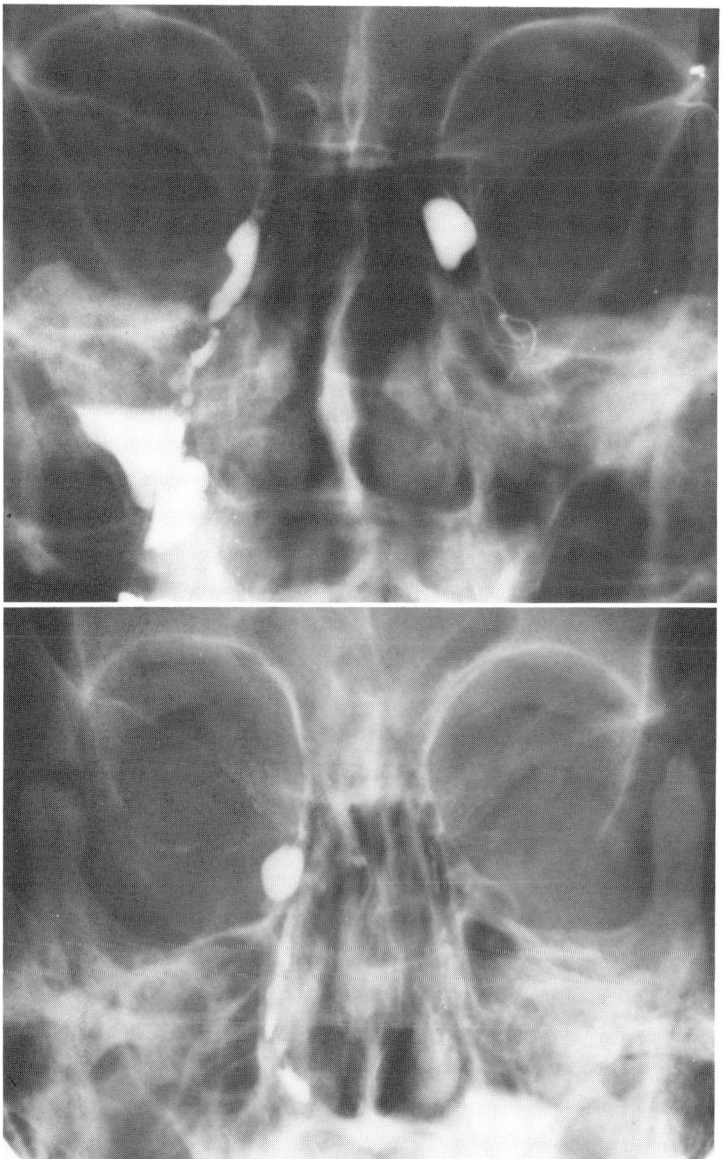

Fig. 8-12. Posttraumatic lacrimal–maxillary antrum fistulas. *Top,* Fistula on right, beginning at junction of lacrimal sac and nasolacrimal junction; there is total obstruction on the left at midsac level. This patient had bilateral dacryocystitis. *Bottom,* Fistula on left was nonsymptomatic. On right, lacrimal sac obstruction caused dacryocystitis; contrast medium could be forced through nasolacrimal duct if injected under slight pressure.

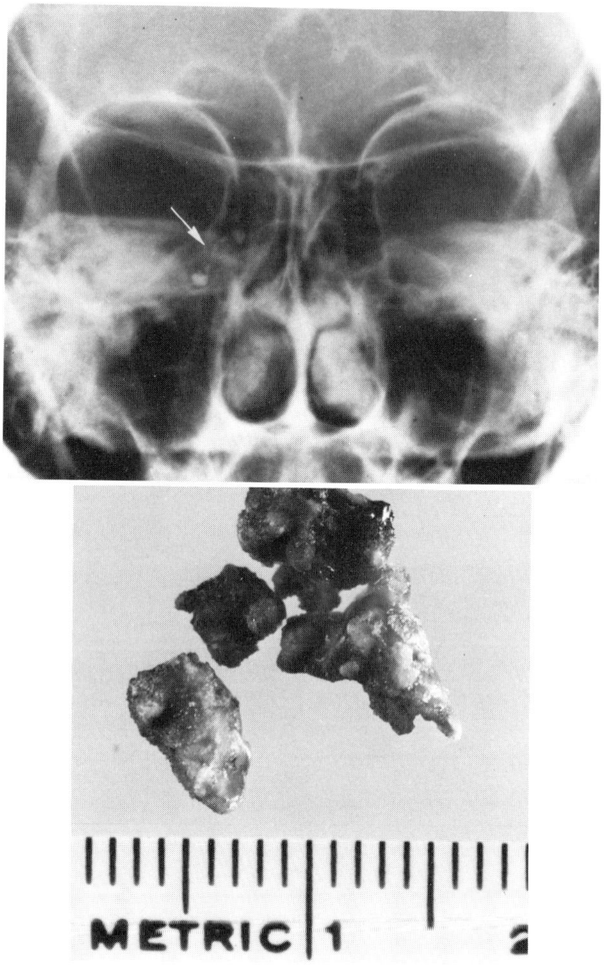

Fig. 8-13. Dacryoliths. *Top,* Markedly irregular outline is seen on roentgenogram after injection of contrast medium. *Bottom,* Multiple soft irregular dacryoliths found at operation.

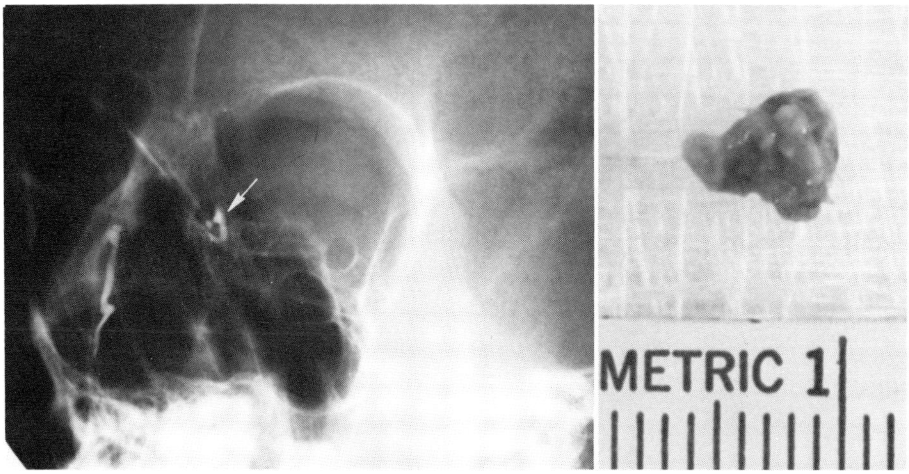

Fig. 8-14. Dacryolith. *Left,* Irregular outline on oblique-view roentgenogram strongly suggests presence of dacryolith. There was obstruction at midsac level. *Right,* Solitary, rough-surfaced dacryolith removed at operation.

dence of a dacryolith. This suspicion is reinforced if the contrast medium can be seen entering the nose, even if injected under mild pressure through the lower punctum while the upper punctum is occluded with a punctal dilator. If the dacryocystogram shows marked irregularity throughout (Fig. 8-13, *top*), multiple soft dacryoliths (Fig. 8-13, *bottom*), usually yellow, may be suspected.

Fig. 8-14 *(left)* demonstrates obstruction at about the middle of the lacrimal sac. The markedly irregular outline suggested a dacryolith, but no fluid could be lavaged into the nose through the canaliculus. The patient had previously undergone dacryocystorhinostomy. At operation the lower half of the lacrimal sac was found to be obstructed by scar tissue; a dacryolith (Fig. 8-14, *right*) filled the upper half of the sac.

When patients have recurrent attacks of acute dacryocystitis, a large, single dacryolith may be blocking both openings into the lacrimal sac (Fig. 8-15). The dacryocystogram may show no abnormal configuration of the sac. If isotonic saline can be lavaged into the nose during the chronic phase of dacryocystitis, the presence of dacryoliths is probable. Occasionally, recurrent acute dacryocystitis will occur with one dacryolith lodged in a pocket at the upper end of the sac while the second dacryolith acts as a ball valve obstructing the entrance into the nasolacrimal duct. The irregular outline seen in Fig. 8-16 suggests the likelihood of a dacryolith; the dacryolith in this case was removed at operation. In a 7-year-old child who began to have acute attacks of dacryocystitis after an automobile accident, an enormously enlarged sac was opened unintentionally during the incision through the skin and deep tissues because the incision was made too laterally (Fig. 8-17).

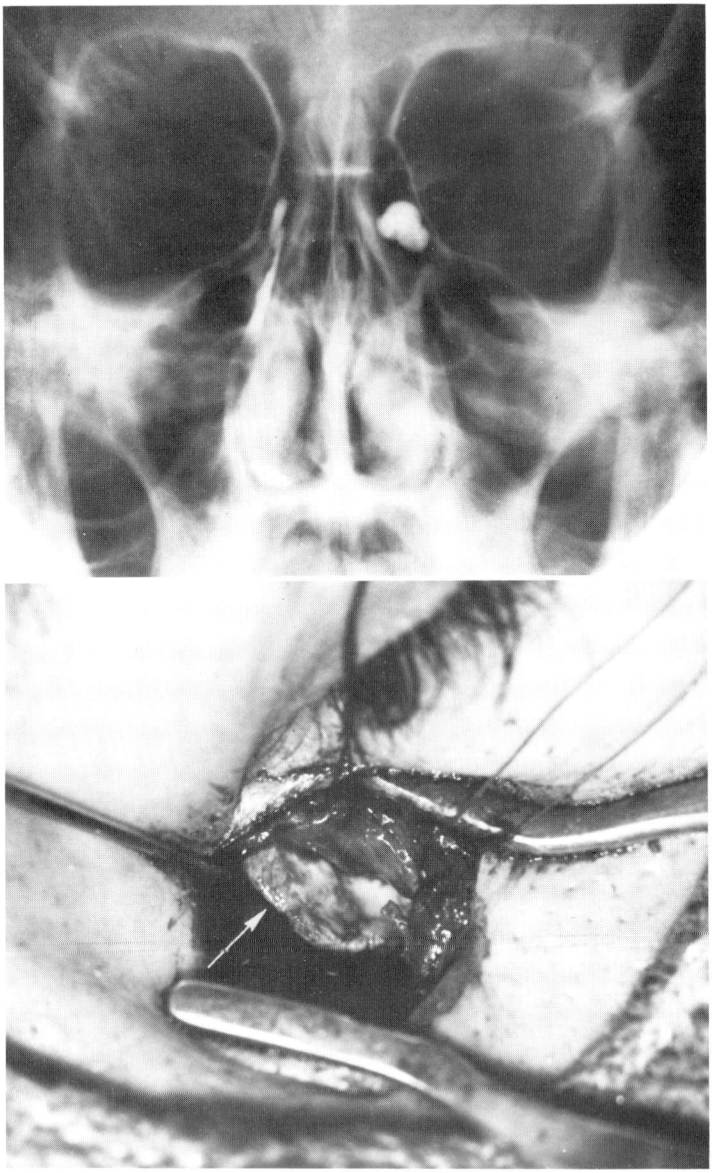

Fig. 8-15. Dacryolith with acute dacryocystitis. *Top,* Dacryocystogram shows irregular outline on left in patient who had recurrent attacks of acute dacryocystitis; obstruction appears to be at midsac level. *Bottom,* At operation, single large "hard" dacryolith is seen filling lacrimal sac.

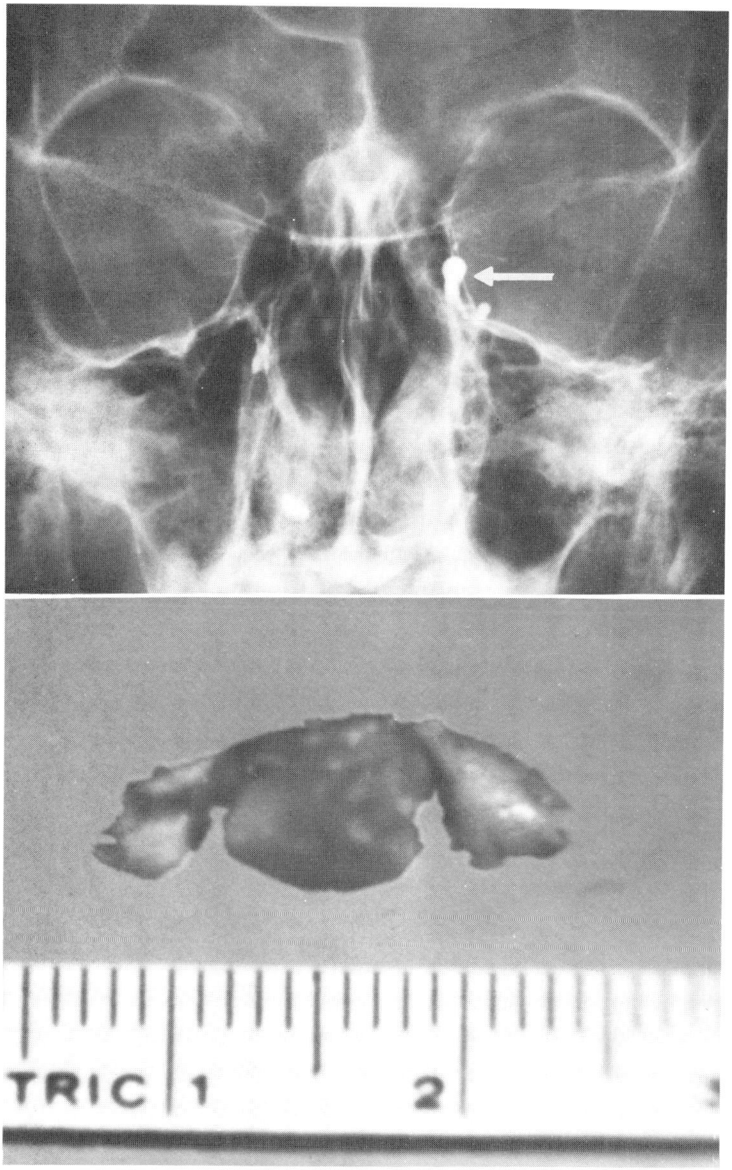

Fig. 8-16. Dacryolith with recurrent acute dacryocystitis. *Top,* Smooth but bizarre outline suggests presence of dacryolith but gives no clue to size or shape. *Bottom,* Operation revealed single dacryolith that almost completely filled dilated lacrimal sac; one end obstructed entrance of common punctum, and other end extended into nasolacrimal duct.

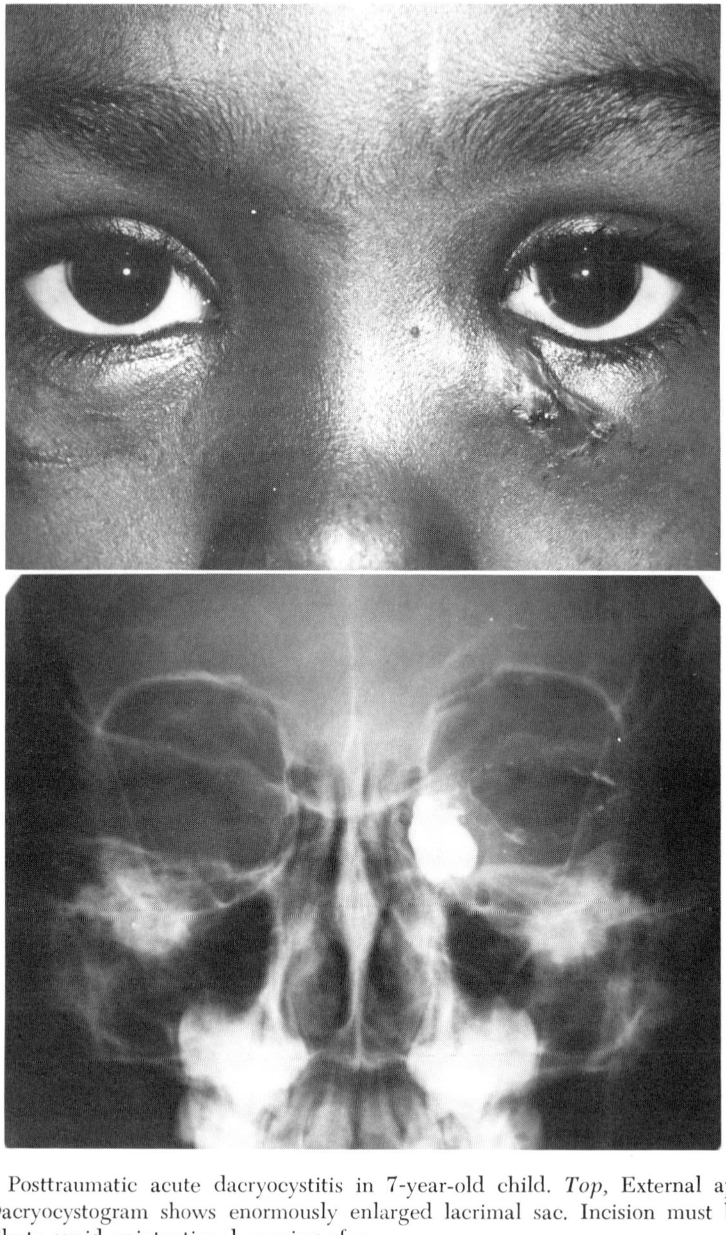

Fig. 8-17. Posttraumatic acute dacryocystitis in 7-year-old child. *Top,* External appearance. *Bottom,* Dacryocystogram shows enormously enlarged lacrimal sac. Incision must be located quite nasally to avoid unintentional opening of sac.

LACRIMAL SAC TUMORS

The diagnosis of lacrimal sac tumor is seldom made by dacryocystography alone. This is because lacrimal sac tumors vary so greatly in size, location, and configuration. The dacryocystograms of lacrimal sacs containing tumors (Fig. 8-18) may closely resemble those of sacs containing dacryoliths. Both are likely to show irregularities in shape and indistinctness in outline. Because lacrimal sac tumors are so rare compared with dacryoliths, the diagnosis is likely to be dacryolith unless other findings are taken into consideration. Fortunately, a mistaken impression of the diagnosis is seldom important. The dacryocystogram will reveal an abnormality, and the patient almost invariably will have signs and symptoms indicating the need for surgical exploration.

Extrinsic tumors may compress the lacrimal sac, preventing tears from draining into the lacrimal sac (Fig. 8-19). Benign tumors of years' duration may show a nondescript irregular outline (Fig. 8-20).

Roentgenograms of lacrimal sacs involved by malignant tumors, like those

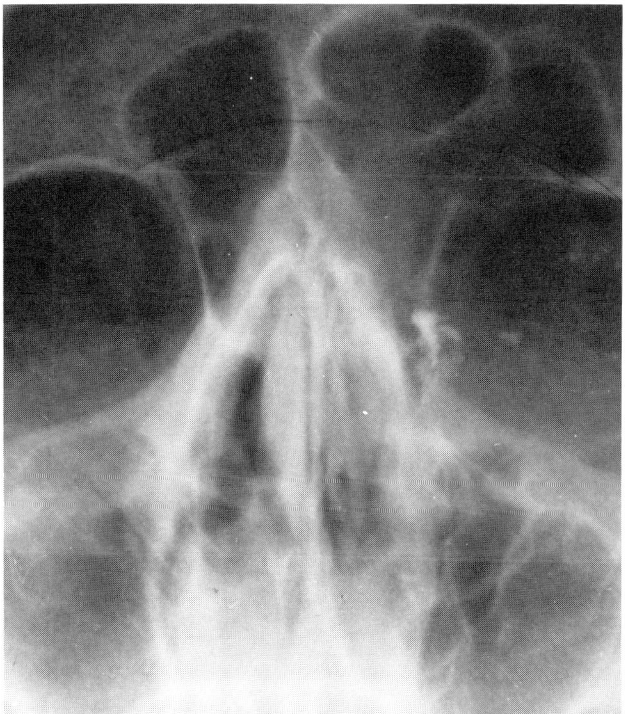

Fig. 8-18. Outline of lacrimal sac is markedly irregular and hazy, suggestive of dacryolith or tumor. Pseudotumor was found at operation.

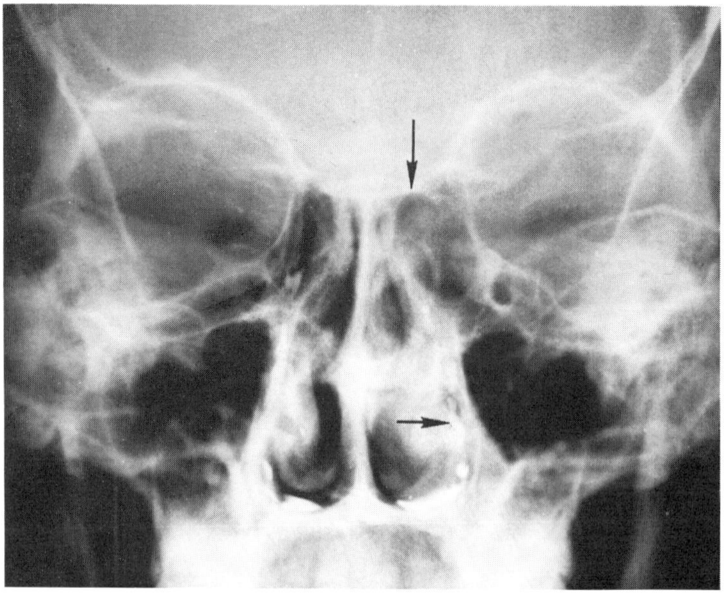

Fig. 8-19. Mucocele *(upper arrow)* compressed lacrimal sac laterally, causing functional obstruction. Contrast medium injected under mild pressure through lower canalicular (with upper punctum occluded) can be seen *(lower arrow)*.

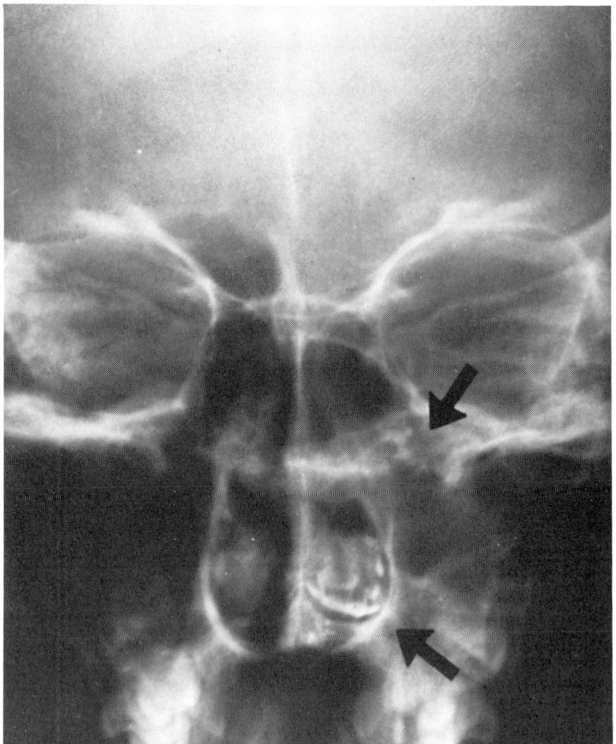

Fig. 8-20. Dacryocystogram shows nondescript, irregular outline of sac and contrast medium in nose in patient with history of allergic rhinitis. At operation, large sac was found filled with friable necrotic tissue and polyps.

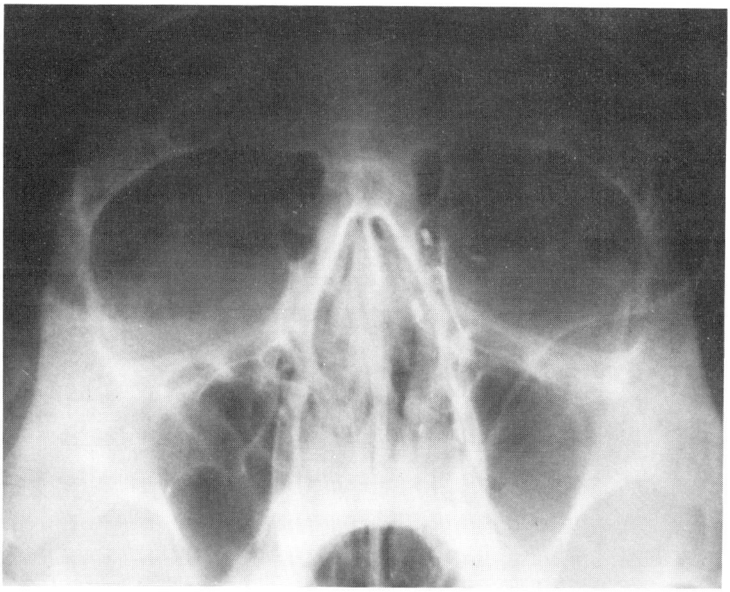

Fig. 8-21. Leukemic infiltrate in patient with chronic lymphocytic leukemia. Contrast medium within sac is scanty and widely distributed.

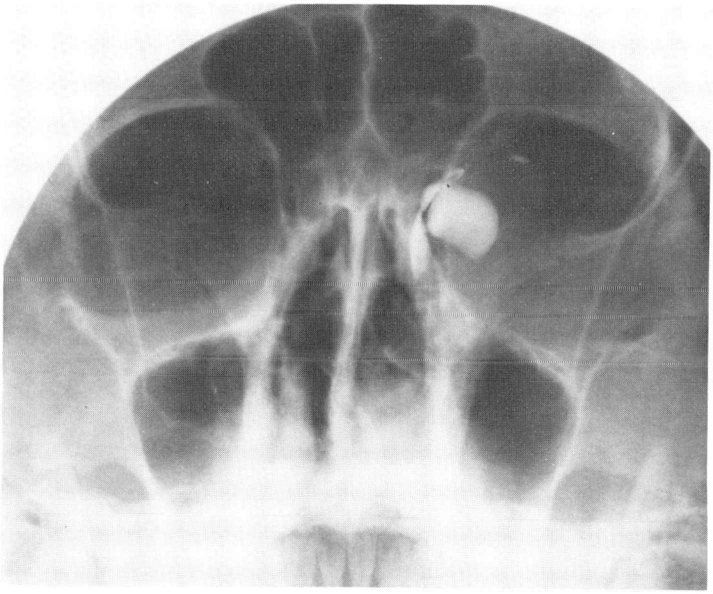

Fig. 8-22. Leiomyosarcoma deforming lacrimal sac. Extensive involvement of all surrounding tissues made it impossible to determine origin of tumor.

of sacs involved by benign tumors, are tremendously varied in their appearance. Dacryocystography will reveal that an abnormality involves the lacrimal sac, but specifics as to the type and extent of the malignancy are determined by surgical exploration and biopsy. In a patient with leukemic involvement the dacryocystogram (Fig. 8-21) suggested only an enlarged sac into which only a minimal amount of radiopaque material could be injected. Extensive involvement of the lacrimal sac and adjacent tissues in a patient with leiomyosarcoma is shown in Fig. 8-22.

The lacrimal drainage system has been studied by use of a technetium-99m lacrimal scan method.[4] Technetium-99m sulfur colloid is placed on each inner margin of the lids, and the radioactively labeled tears are traced with a gamma camera as they flow down the lacrimal drainage system. Preliminary studies suggest that this technique is excellent for determining the status of the tear drainage. The biggest disadvantage would seem to be the expense of the equipment—about $50,000—which would limit its availability. Whether this method will have a significant advantage over established methods, such as the dye test, dacryocystography, and other tests, remains to be seen.

REFERENCES

1. Gerlock, A. J., Jr.: A simple radiographic technic for visualization of the lacrimal foramen, South Med J 68:118-120, 1975.
2. Lloyd, G. A. S., Jones, B. R., and Welham, R. A. N.: Intubation macrodacryocystography, Br J Ophthalmol 56:600-603, 1972.
3. Putterman, A. M.: Dacryocystography with occluded common canaliculus, Am J Ophthalmol 76:1010-1011, 1973.
4. Saparoff, G., Chaudhuri, T. K., Chaudhuri, T. K., Dolan, K., and Christie, J. H.: Contrast dacryocystography vs. technetium-99m lacrimal scan. Read at the 80th annual meeting of the American Academy of Ophthalmology and Otolaryngology, Dallas, Texas, Sept. 21-25, 1975.

CHAPTER 9

Lacrimal sac surgery: external dacryocystorhinostomy

HISTORY

Procedures for correction of disorders of the lacrimal sac date back more than 2,000 years. Picó[5] has described the development of different techniques of dacryocystorhinostomy. Present-day techniques stem from the Toti procedure, which he reported[6] in 1904.

ANATOMIC CONSIDERATIONS

A knowledge of the anatomy of the medial palpebral tendon is tremendously important to anyone doing lacrimal surgery. Its position can be instantly detected. Because the orbicularis oculi muscles have their origins in the tendon, secure replacement of it is mandatory if the tendon is avulsed or severed.

This tendon of tough connective tissue originates from the superior portion of the frontal process of the maxilla. The anterior part of the tendon takes its origin from the upper several millimeters of the anterior lacrimal crest. The origin also extends in an anteromedial direction as far as the nasomaxillary suture. The superior border of the tendon is continuous with the periosteum of the frontal process of the maxilla. The lower border of the tendon is free. This explains why during acute or subacute dacryocystitis the swelling of the lacrimal sac is confined to the area below the tendon. Swelling will extend above the tendon in some cases of lacrimal sac tumor.

The angular vessels cross anteriorly to the tendon, about 3 mm medially to the inner canthus. These vessels run in a curved course, convexity outward. In making an incision into the lacrimal sac, it is difficult to avoid cutting the vessels or the larger branches. Hemostasis is simple. Usually, the bleeding vessels are clamped with a hemostat, and a diathermy tip (with the patient grounded) is applied to the hemostat.

In most cases the lacrimal sac extends only about 2 mm superiorly to the tendon, not the 4 mm or so commonly mentioned. This makes swinging the dome of the sac into the lacrimal lake region somewhat difficult.

It is totally unnecessary to sever the tendon in a routine external dacryocystorhinostomy. Carrying the anastomosis that high is undesirable because (1) it may damage the common canaliculus, which empties into the sac posteriorly; (2) ethmoid cells usually are encountered if anastomosis is carried that high; (3) it may damage the tendon; (4) ample room is available inferiorly to the tendon for a sufficiently large anastomosis; and (5) a bowstring or webbing type of scar is more likely to result if the incision includes the tendon. Severing the medial palpebral tendon is justifiable in a few instances. Generally, the intact tendon serves as a superb landmark for making the incision as well as for performing most of the operation.

PROGNOSIS

The incidence of permanent relief of symptoms in patients with acute or chronic dacryocystitis is nearly 100% in routine cases. The most favorable cases are those in which the lacrimal sac is large and has no other pathologic condition. The less favorable cases are those with (1) scarring in and around the lacrimal sac due to trauma or previous operations, (2) a small lacrimal sac, (3) nasal disorders such as nasal polyps or markedly deviated nasal septum toward the side to be operated on, and (4) a tumor or constriction involving the sac or canaliculi.

The outlook for relief of symptoms in the unfavorable cases has improved substantially with improvement in technique. Usually, a successful anastomosis with the nose can be accomplished so long as a remnant of the lacrimal sac remains. The favorable prognosis of a properly performed external dacryocystorhinostomy has relegated removal of the lacrimal sac to the status of an exceptionally rare procedure, malignancy involving the sac being about the only indication for it.

External dacryocystorhinostomy has almost completely supplanted the intranasal approach. The intranasal approach is technically different. A large anastomosis cannot be made, and inspection of the sac for disorders such as tumors or dacryoliths is less than satisfactory.

Intubation of the nasolacrimal duct, either via the canaliculi and sac or retrograde from the nose, has not proved to be a successful substitute for the external approach. Only in the very young (for example, those with dacryocystitis secondary to congenital occlusion of the nasolacrimal duct that does not respond to probing) would intubation be considered at all as a substitute to the external approach. Injury to the canaliculi is common when intubation is attempted through them. Dacryoliths, tumors, and other disorders of the lacrimal sac would be complicating factors.

In summary, the prognosis in the majority of patients treated with a properly performed external dacryocystorhinostomy is exceptionally good. Except for probing in the very young, other techniques have marginal value.

INDICATIONS

Dacryocystorhinostomy is indicated for most patients with dacryocystitis. Probing of the nasolacrimal duct will cure dacryocystitis in nearly 100% of patients less than 1 year old and in many between the ages of 1 and 2 years. In patients older than this, probing of the nasolacrimal duct is not only painful but is much more likely to aggravate the problem than to improve it, yet many ophthalmologists continue the probing until the patient (usually) calls a halt.

In the young, dacryocystorhinostomy should be postponed until about age 3 years. By this time the structures are larger, making the operation easier, and general anesthesia is perhaps safer. Except for the parents' having to put up with a "messy eye," no disadvantages are likely from this wait.

Adult patients, even those in their 80s if in reasonably good health, may be relieved of annoying and at times painful symptoms in instances of acute dacryocystitis.

An external dacryocystorhinostomy should be performed to relieve lacrimal sac infection prior to intraocular surgery; dacryocystectomy should never be substituted because, at best, tear stasis will persist. More importantly, in approximately one third of the patients who undergo dacryocystectomy, part of the sac mucosa is left behind and a new lacrimal sac forms.

Borderline situations occur, for example, when the nasolacrimal duct is completely and permanently blocked but infection is minimal. The younger the patient, the more likely that tear secretion will be greater, causing a more annoying epiphora. Also, because of longer life expectancy, troublesome infection usually will develop sooner or later.

Failures from previous dacryocystorhinostomy or attempted dacryocystectomy are not necessarily a contraindication to the operation because most failures can be turned into successes. If intranasal pathologic conditions exist (although they are relatively infrequent) that might contribute to the failure of dacryocystorhinostomy, these conditions should be corrected as far as possible before lacrimal surgery is undertaken. Nasal polyps, nasal allergies, severely deviated nasal septum (toward the side to be operated on), and sinusitis are some of the more frequently encountered nasal conditions that may require treatment.

Failure to diagnose the patient's lacrimal drainage system disorder properly may condemn the patient to endure annoying symptoms that could be easily corrected by an external dacryocystorhinostomy. For example, the ophthalmologist may be able to irrigate fluid into the nose with symptoms suggestive of dacryocystitis and decide that no pathologic condition of the sac exists. In many instances such patients have dacryoliths, lacrimal sac tumors, or functional occlusion of the nasolacrimal duct. Dacryocystography (see Chapter 8) offers invaluable aid in determining whether the operation is indicated.

CONTRAINDICATIONS

Malignant involvement of the lacrimal sac is the prime contraindication to dacryocystorhinostomy. These cases are rare, and often the diagnosis is not made until the lacrimal sac is exposed. If the lacrimal sac contains a benign neoplasm, polyps, or granuloma, the prognosis is less bright, but these circumstances are not contraindications to the operation.

Age per se is seldom a contraindication to the performance of a dacryocystorhinostomy. I prefer to wait until young patients are about 3 years old. I have performed the operation many times in patients in their 80s without untoward results. Elderly patients with minimal symptoms from lacrimal sac infections may prefer to live with their condition rather than have a surgical correction. A dacryocystorhinostomy is usually contraindicated when life expectancy is short. Removal of the lacrimal sac should not be substituted for a dacryocystorhinostomy because removal of the sac is a major procedure that frequently leaves the patient with annoying symptoms.

Atrophy of the lacrimal sac has been mentioned as a contraindication to dacryocystorhinostomy. Whether a sac is atrophic is difficult to determine preoperatively and probably has little if anything to do with the success of the operation. Weakness of the orbicularis oculi muscles, ectropion of the lower punctum, or partial stenosis of the canaliculi would seem a more likely cause for failure, especially failure to relieve the epiphora. If the anastomosis between the lacrimal sac and the nose is adequate, the dacryocystitis will almost certainly be cured.

ANESTHESIA

Whether local or general anesthesia is used depends on many factors, such as age of the patient, general condition (and often the patient's preference), and the experience of the operator. General anesthesia should be used for most patients under the age of 16 to 18 years and for the highly apprehensive patient. While some experienced surgeons prefer to use general anesthesia for all lacrimal sac operations, I prefer to use local anesthesia for adults except for the highly nervous patient. The risk in performing the operation under local anesthesia is minimal in the elderly or in those who may have circulatory or other conditions that might make general anesthesia hazardous.

Local anesthesia

Preoperative steps. The patient is hospitalized on the day prior to the operation and medication, including a hypnotic agent to ensure a good night's sleep, is administered as indicated. Administration of pentobarbital sodium (Nembutal), 40 to 50 mg, and meperidine hydrochloride (Demerol), 40 to 100 mg, 1 hour preoperatively will usually ensure that the patient is well sedated. If the patient is particularly apprehensive during any part of the operative procedure, diazepam (Valium), 5 to 10 mg intramuscularly (or intravenously), or an additional dose of meperidine may simplify matters for the patient and the surgeon. An antiemetic agent also may be indicated preoperatively.

Technique. A vasoconstricting solution such as phenylephrine hydrochloride (Neo-Synephrine hydrochloride, 0.25%) may be sprayed into the nose on the side to be operated on or both sides if both are to be operated on using a hand-operated nebulizer and a rubber bulb. The tip of the nebulizer should be pointed anteriorly and superiorly so that the nasal mucosa adjacent to the lacrimal sac is sprayed. The nose is sprayed shortly thereafter with a topical anesthetic such as tetracaine hydrochloride (Pontocaine hydrochloride, 2%).

To prolong the effect of the nasal medication, a thin pledget of cotton about 5 cm long is saturated with the topical anesthetic agent, the excess fluid is squeezed out, and the pledget is inserted into the nose with a nasal applicator. Practice is required to enable the ophthalmologist to use a head mirror for placement of the cotton pledget as far anteriorly and superiorly as possible (in the area where the anastomosis from the lacrimal sac into the nose will be made later). Many residents will force a large wad of cotton into the nose in the wrong position. A postnasal pack to prevent aspiration of blood or mucus is unnecessary.

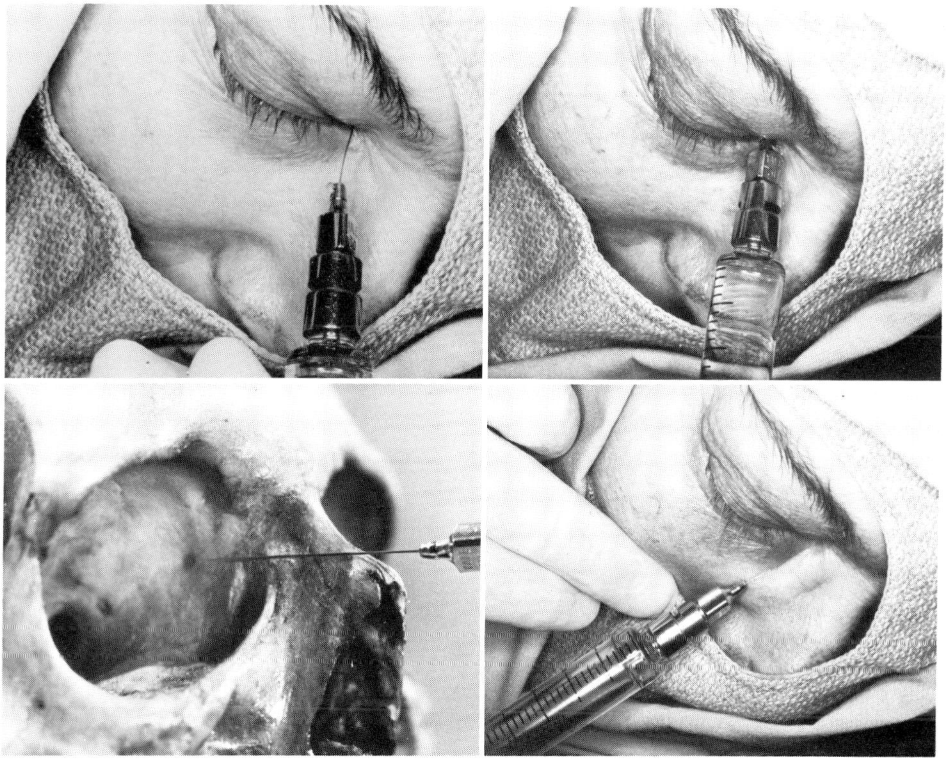

A B C D

Fig. 9-1. Procedure for local anesthesia. **A,** Beginning injection of nasociliary nerve. The 30-gauge needle is directed posteriorly in horizontal position. Needle enters soft tissue immediately superior to medial palpebral tendon and is directed to follow medial bony orbital wall. **B,** Injection of nasociliary nerve. Medial orbital tissues are injected as needle is slowly passed posteriorly, 20 to 25 mm. **C,** Course of needle, showing its tip reaching the anterior ethmoid foramen. **D,** Use of 30-gauge needle to infiltrate anesthetic agent into soft tissues overlying lacrimal sac region. (**C** from Veirs, E.: Appropriate anesthesia. In Veirs, E.: The lacrimal system: Proceedings of the first international symposium, St. Louis, 1970, The C. V. Mosby Co., pp. 133-136.)

The side (or sides) to be operated on are then scrubbed and draped. Blocking of the anterior ethmoid nerve and the infratrochlear branches of the nasociliary nerve with an anesthetic agent greatly facilitates development of good anesthesia. The anterior ethmoid nerve supplies much of the interior of the nose involved in the operation. The infratrochlear nerve supplies the skin and conjunctiva at the inner canthal region, lacrimal sac, canaliculi, and caruncle.

A 30-gauge needle is attached to a 2-ml syringe that contains an anesthetic agent such as lidocaine (Xylocaine, 2%). The needle is directed posteriorly in a horizontal plane to enter the orbit just above the medial palpebral tendon. The solution is slowly injected as the needle passes posteriorly about 20 mm, hugging the medial bony wall of the orbit. About 1 ml of the anesthetic agent is injected. This blocks the anterior ethmoid as well as the inferior trochlear nerve (Fig. 9-1, *A* to *C*). The only side effect I have encountered from this nerve block is temporary diplopia from paralysis of the medial rectus muscle, and this occurred only when the injection was given prior to an office procedure on the lacrimal system. An additional 2 ml of the anesthetic agent is injected in the region of the lacrimal sac (Fig. 9-1, *D*).

General anesthesia

The anesthesiologist should be informed that nasal bleeding may be sufficient to cause significant amounts of blood to enter the lungs unless measures are taken to prevent this. Some anesthesiologists insert sufficiently large intratracheal breathing tubes in the very young to prevent blood from entering the trachea. Intratracheal cuffs also are used frequently for this purpose.

OPERATIVE PROCEDURE

Skin incision

The skin incision begins about 3 mm medially to the inner canthus and just inferior to the medial palpebral tendon and is carried downward in a nearly straight line for about 25 mm. No attempt is made to follow the curve of the anterior lacrimal crest as the incision is carried inferiorly. To do so will result in a curved incision that often forms a bowstring scar. This first bold stroke should include all the soft tissues down to the bone (Fig. 9-2).

If the patient has a greatly enlarged lacrimal sac, the incision should be made more nasally to avoid entering the sac unintentionally. The angular vessels may be avoided if the original incision is made 4 to 5 mm medially to the inner canthus. The disadvantage is that access to the lacrimal sac is more difficult because the soft tissues must be retracted further laterally. There is no advantage in including the medial palpebral tendon in the incision in routine cases.

Bleeding may be profuse as the original incision is completed, especially if the operation is performed under general anesthesia. If a spurting blood vessel is seen, it may be clamped before the speculum is inserted. Good suction is

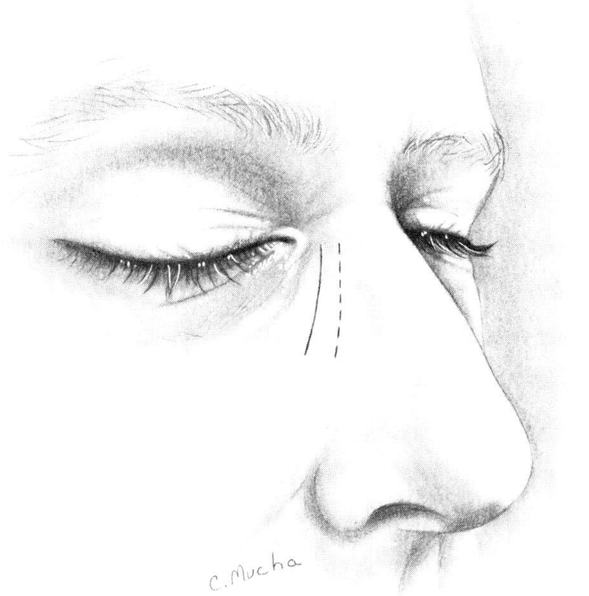

Fig. 9-2. Skin incision is carried inferiorly through all soft tissues in one cut. Optimal curve usually results without intentional effort. More medial incision *(interrupted line)* is used to avoid unintentionally entering a large lacrimal sac.

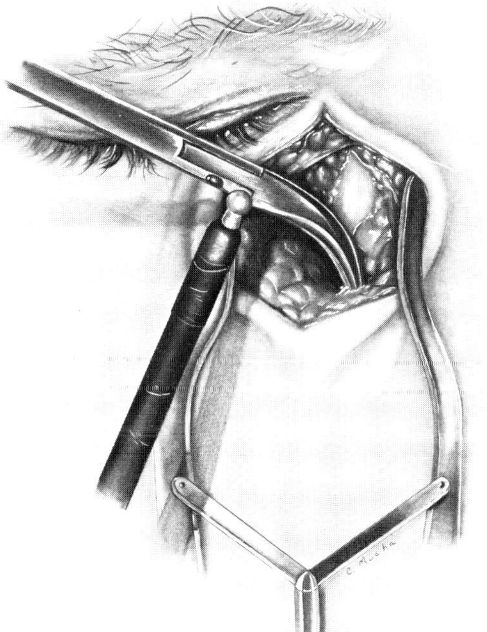

Fig. 9-3. Hemostat clamping bleeding vessels is touched with diathermy cautery tip (patient is grounded). Care must be taken not to touch tissue except where cauterization is intended.

necessary. Immediate insertion of the lacrimal speculum may slow the bleeding appreciably. The vessels are clamped with a small, curved hemostat. With the patient grounded, the hemostat is touched with the tip of a ball-point cautery (Fig. 9-3). This quickly and effectively closes the bleeding vessels.

Often, an annoying bleeding point is encountered where a small vessel exits from the bone, 3 or 4 mm medially to the anterior lacrimal crest and toward the inferior portion of the exposed bone. This bleeding can easily be stopped by applying diathermy with a ball-point tip. Strong cautery may be used if needed because this bone will later be removed.

Exposure of lacrimal sac

The original incision will expose the bone 3 mm or so medially to the anterior lacrimal crest. This bone is the frontal process of the maxilla and usually is relatively thick. The periosteum is separated from the bone medially and laterally to the anterior lacrimal crest with a Freer periosteal elevator. In a

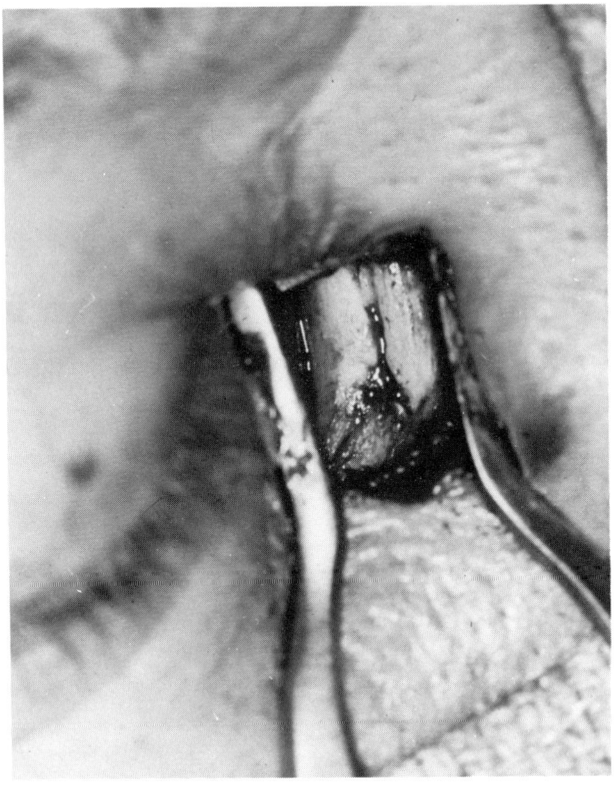

Fig. 9-4. Prominent sutura notha. Medially, the anterior lacrimal crest is rounded. An annoying bleeder may exit within this suture or at this area in more routine-appearing bone. A small ball-point diathermy cautery applied directly to bleeding point in bone will stop bleeding.

few instances the sutura notha, a bony groove that runs parallel and 3 or 4 mm medially to the anterior lacrimal crest, is quite prominent (Fig. 9-4). This groove may be confused at first with the anterior lacrimal crest. At this point the periosteum adheres more tightly to the bone, and care must be taken not to injure the lacrimal sac. The anterior lacrimal crest is the important landmark in locating the sac—the sac lies in the lacrimal fossa that is lateral and posterior to the anterior lacrimal crest. The lacrimal sac enclosed in the periosteum is readily identified by its smooth, light gray appearance (Fig. 9-5). The sac can be easily separated from its medial bony wall and retracted laterally with a Freer elevator.

Bony anastomosis

The bone that separates the lacrimal sac from the nasal mucosa is now removed (Fig. 9-6). The technique used for this should be the one best suited to the operator. The important considerations are (1) making the bony opening large (about 15 mm vertically and 8 mm horizontally but smaller in young children), (2) placing the opening in an anteroinferior position, (3) avoiding damage to the lacrimal sac and nasal mucosa or other structures.

I prefer to use a dental drill with about a 3-mm-diameter bur to remove most

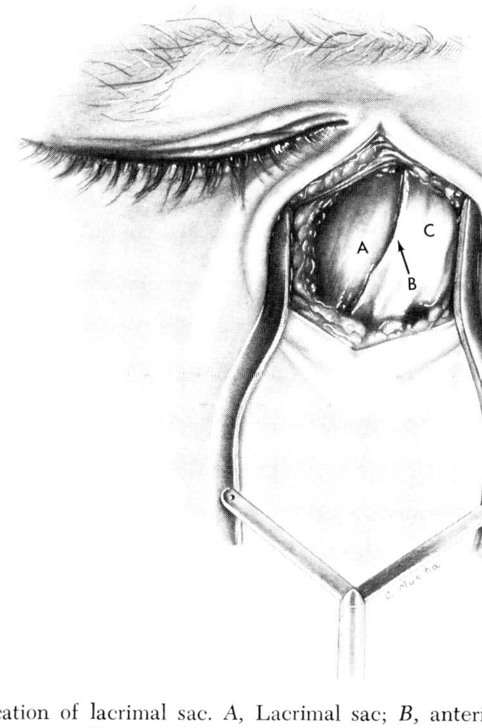

Fig. 9-5. Identification of lacrimal sac. *A*, Lacrimal sac; *B*, anterior lacrimal crest; *C*, frontal process of maxilla. Exposed bone plus most of lacrimal bone will be removed.

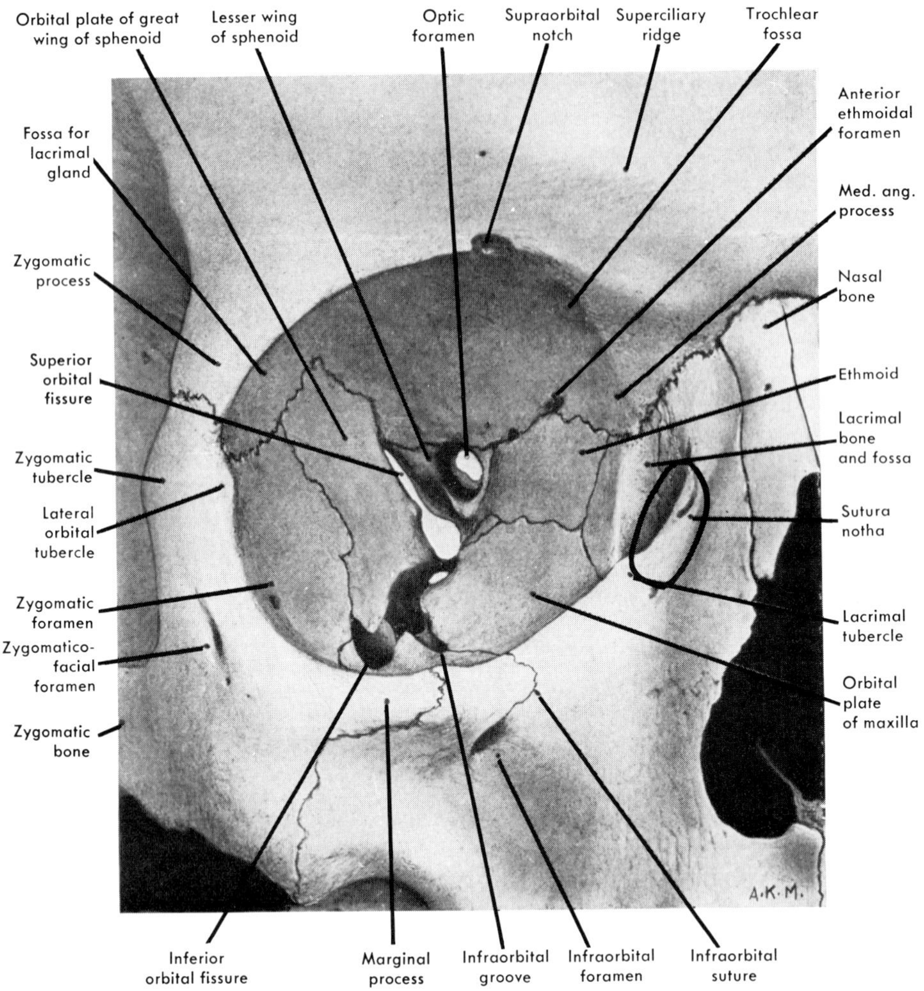

Fig. 9-6. Approximate area of bone removed in adults to create anastomosis. (From Last, R. J.: Wolff's Anatomy of the eye and orbit, ed. 3, Toronto, 1948, The Blakiston Company.)

of the bone (Fig. 9-7). Drills driven electrically (Jordan Day, manufactured by Zimmer) or by air or nitrous oxide (Stryker or Hall, manufactured by Minnesota Mining and Manufacturing Co.) are satisfactory. The handle of the drill should be held with both hands to keep it under control, usually with the right hand resting on the patient's draped face. The drilling may be begun 2 or 3 mm medially to the exposed anterior lacrimal crest. Some time is required to expose the nasal mucosa if the bone is hard and thick. Great care must be taken not to damage the nasal mucosa as the bone is removed; the intact mucosa may be essential to the success of the operation.

A Freer elevator inserted between the sac and the bone is helpful in pro-

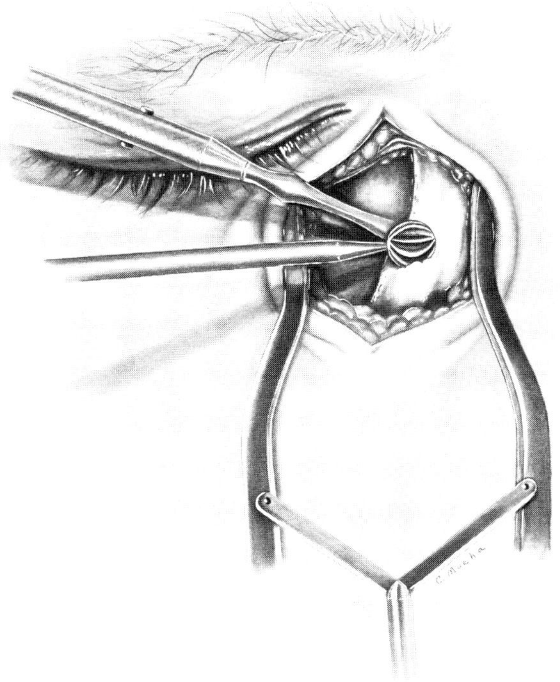

Fig. 9-7. Dental drill used to remove bone to expose nasal mucosa. Further bone removal can be accomplished with bone-biting forceps or the bur or both. Freer elevator is used to protect lacrimal sac.

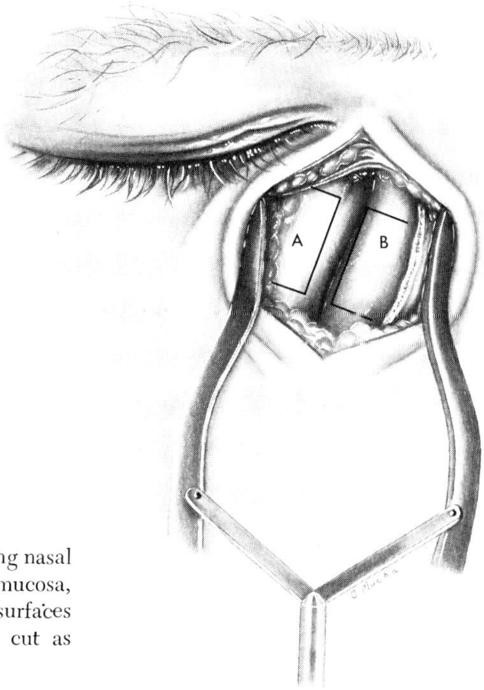

Fig. 9-8. Large bony opening, exposing nasal wall of lacrimal sac, *A*, and nasal mucosa, *B*. Posteriorly, the two mucosal surfaces meet in a V. Membranous flaps are cut as outlined by black lines.

tecting the sac mucosa. An assistant irrigates with isotonic saline intermittently and manages the suction as well, using the Frazier suction tip.

After sufficient bone is removed by the drill, an Adler punch forceps is useful to enlarge the opening enough to allow a more powerful bone-biting instrument (Kerrison rongeur, size 0) to be used. A Lampert straight rongeur is useful in removing the more posteriorly placed lacrimal bone. The bony opening can be started by the use of other instruments such as a trephine or chisel.

The important considerations are to make the opening large enough and in the correct position without damaging the nasal mucosa. In adults the bony opening should extend inferiorly for about 15 mm, starting from about 2 mm inferior to the medial palpebral tendon. This will include the superior medial portion of the bony nasolacrimal duct, allowing a larger membranous anastomosis into the nose to be established. Posteriorly, the bone should be removed until the nasal and lacrimal sac mucosas seem to join, although they are actually separated by the very thin plate (Fig. 9-8). Removal of an adequate amount of bone will allow for a large anastomosis from the lacrimal sac into the nose, ensuring a high percentage of permanent cures.

Making a large bony anastomosis is especially helpful in cases with a less favorable prognosis, for example, those with small lacrimal sacs or markedly scarred tissues. This allows a large amount of nasal mucosa to partly compensate for the smaller amount of lacrimal sac mucosa when the membranous anastomosis is fashioned. Generous removal of bone in an anteroinferior direction is important because this allows the anastomosis to be made in the middle meatus of the bone. The ethmoid air cells are adjacent to the upper half of the lacrimal fossa. The medial palpebral tendon is a key landmark in removing bone as well as in fashioning the membranous flaps. Limiting the operative procedure to the area inferior to this tendon should prevent damage to the common punctum.

Occasionally, annoying bleeding points will be seen in the exposed nasal mucosa. The small ball-point diathermy tip can be used to stop this bleeding instantly.

Mucosal incisions

Care should be taken to properly identify the lacrimal sac and to fashion flaps that will provide the largest anastomosis possible. A large bony opening will facilitate this step. When the sac is small or is involved by extensive scarring from previous operations or injury, passing a no. 0 or 1 Bowman probe through the lower or upper canaliculus to "tent" the lacrimal sac medially helps in its identification (Fig. 9-9). If the scarring is severe, the probe will not tent the sac. Careful dissection of the area with long-handled Stevens scissors until the probe that has been passed into the sac is exposed is the most satisfactory method of identifying the sac.

Quadrangular flaps of both lacrimal sac and nasal mucosa, hinged anteriorly, are easy to fashion and help provide a large anastomosis between the sac and

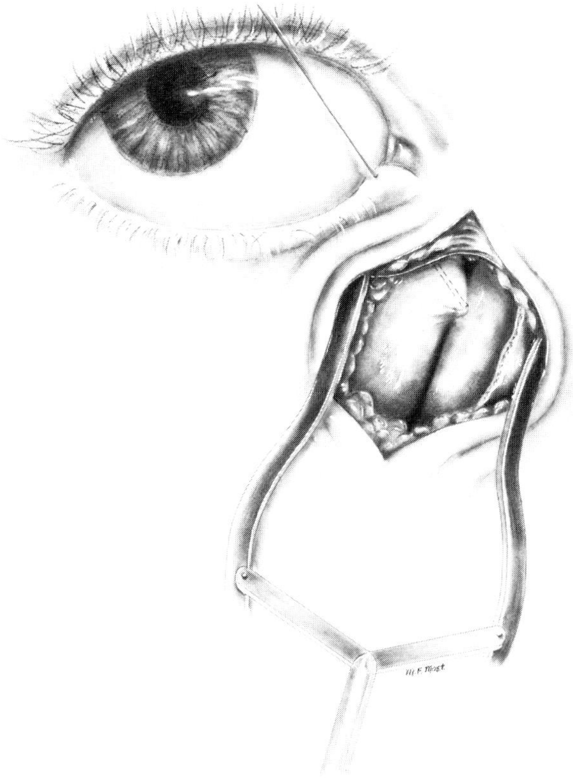

Fig. 9-9. Lacrimal probe passed through canaliculus "tents" sac to help identify it. Identifying probe within sac after sac is opened may be useful.

the nose. A no. 11 Bard-Parker blade is useful for incision of the sac and nasal mucosa from an anteroposterior direction. The posterior borders of the flaps are often more easily incised with small scissors (such as Stevens scissors) with a long handle. Because the bleeding from it is less, the flap of sac mucosa is fashioned first. A suture of 4-0 catgut with a small half-circle needle (no. 10352-33, Davis & Geck Division, American Cyanamid Company) is then passed through the upper edge of the incised lacrimal flap, and another is passed through the lower edge of the incised nasal mucosa, or vice versa. The sutures can then be used to hold the flaps laterally so that the interior of the sac can be inspected (Fig. 9-10).

The sac is then inspected carefully for dacryoliths, tumors, and other problems. If any doubt exists that the common canaliculus is stenosed, it is well to irrigate isotonic saline through the canaliculi. Hecht[2] recommends following the saline injection with air injection if difficulty is encountered in identifying the common punctum. If there is a pathologic condition in the region of the common canaliculus, careful exposure of this region of the sac is indicated. (Re-

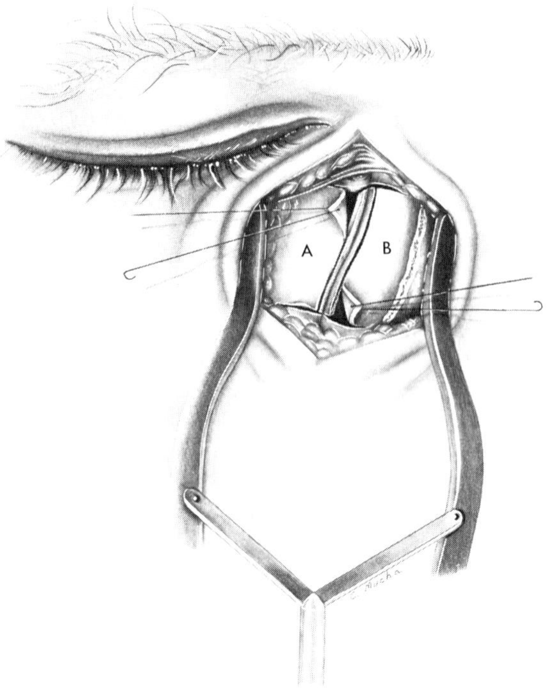

Fig. 9-10. Membranous flaps have been incised and sutures are in place before cautery. Traction on sutures exposes inside of sac and nose for inspection. Pulling membrane apart also allows posterior and inferior lips of wound to be cauterized. (*A*, lacrimal sac mucosa; *B*, nasal mucosa.)

member that the opening of the common canaliculus into the sac is at the level of the medial palpebral tendon.)

When dacryoliths are present, they block the spontaneous flow of tears into the nose. After removal of the dacryoliths the drainage passages will almost always be found patent; however, the routine dacryocystorhinostomy should always be performed when dacryoliths are present because otherwise the dacryoliths may recur. The prognosis is exceptionally good in these cases because the patient is left with a large anastomosis from the sac into the nose as well as with a patent nasolacrimal duct.

Occasionally, nasal polyps or nasal obstructions (Fig. 9-11) may come into excellent view. It usually is preferable to have this type of abnormality corrected by an otolaryngologist prior to the lacrimal surgery. Polyps and other nasal pathologic conditions may be corrected through the newly formed nasal opening. This procedure is sometimes combined with the external nares approach. Unfortunately, most ophthalmologists may feel they are lacking in the expertise needed to deal with the more complicated situations properly. If, by its position or size, a portion of turbinate appears likely to compromise the

A

B

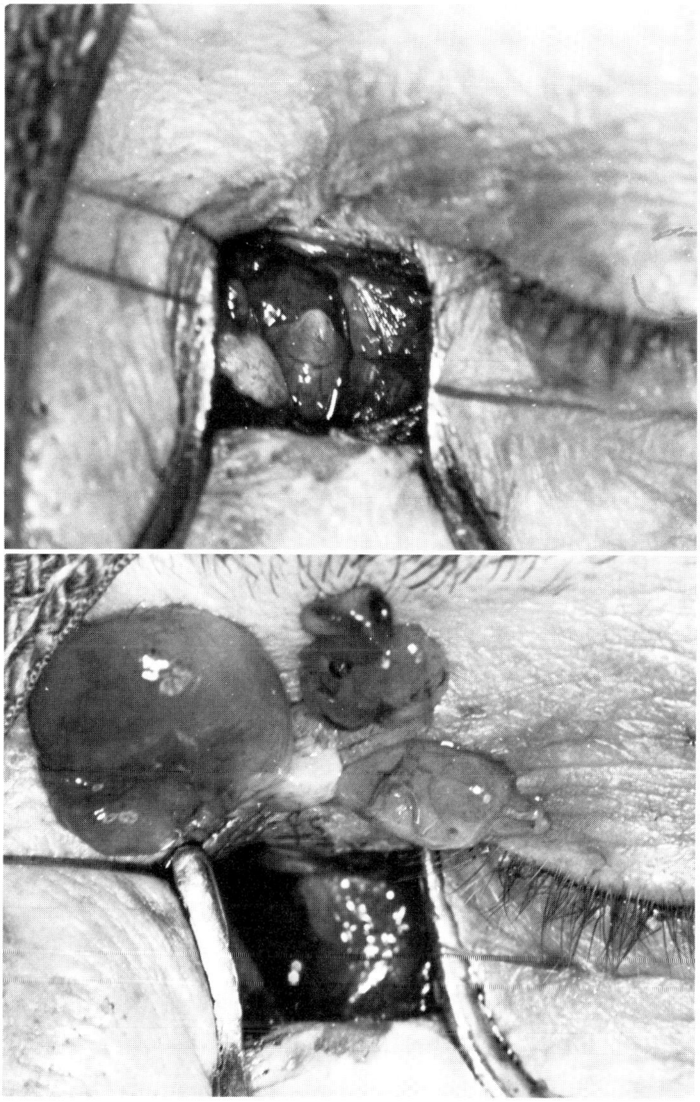

Fig. 9-11. Nasal polyps. **A,** After nasal and lacrimal sac mucosas are incised, polyps can be seen filling nose. **B,** Polyps removed through newly formed opening and by conventional approach through external nares.

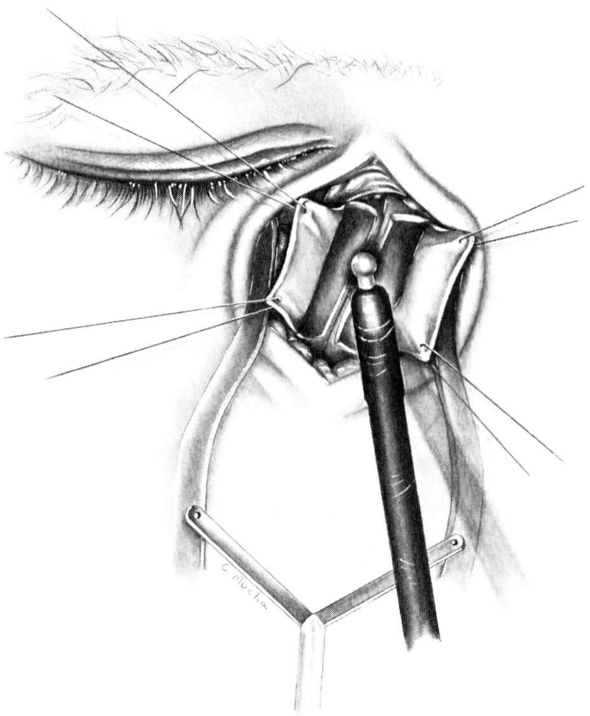

Fig. 9-12. With nasal and lacrimal sac membranous flaps held aside, diathermy cautery is used to thoroughly cauterize posterior and inferior cut edges of anastomosis. This greatly enlarges size of anastomosis. Care should be taken not to damage common punctum by cauterizing too far superiorly.

anastomosis, that portion should be removed. This is easily accomplished with an ethmoid cup forceps through the newly formed opening into the nose.

Cauterization of lips of anastomosis

With the nasal and sac mucosas held in opposite directions, the posterior and inferior lips of the anastomosis opening are cauterized with a ball-point cautery (Fig. 9-12). The cauterizing current may have to be increased some for this procedure.

Without cauterization it is difficult if not impossible to make the membranous opening as large as the bony anastomosis. Also, it is possible that the cauterization helps to prevent closure of the anastomosis. The need for hemostasis may be decreased after the cauterization. Unfortunately, some patients will experience some pain from the cautery in an otherwise painless operation.

Suturing

The procedure for fashioning and suturing the anterior and posterior mucosal flaps is difficult. This is especially true if the lacrimal sac is small or scarred.

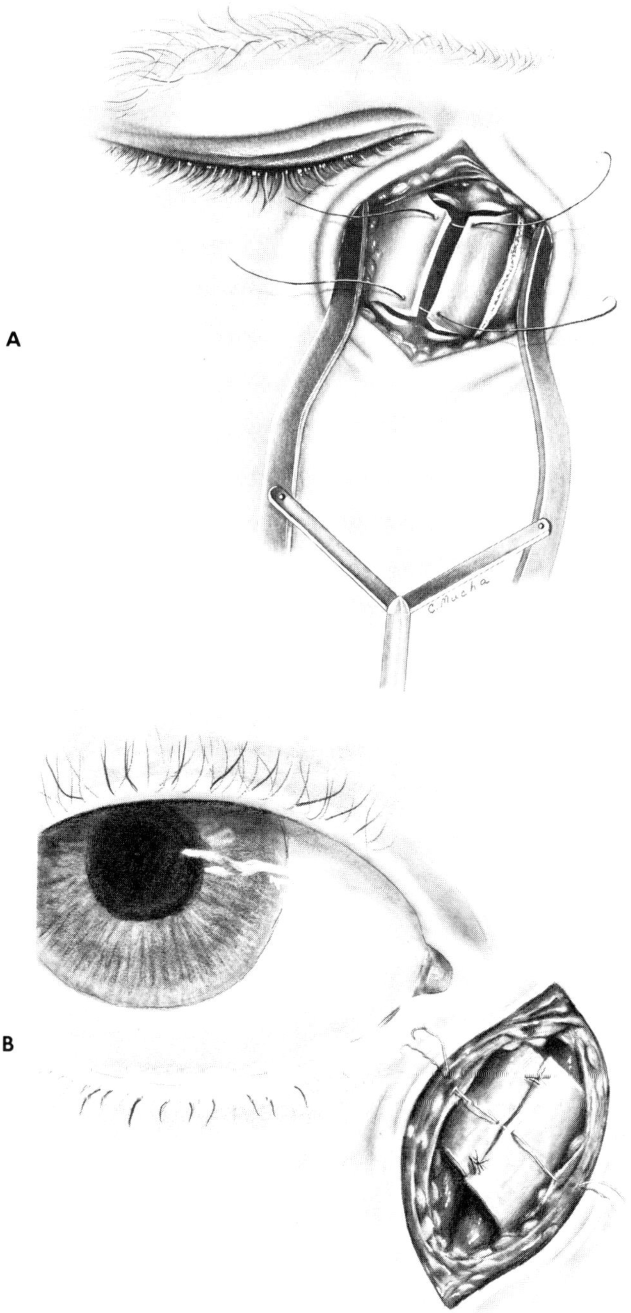

Fig. 9-13. Suturing. **A,** Mucosal flaps, hinged anteriorly, being sutured together. **B,** Suture holding flap forward.

When the lacrimal sac is large, the prognosis should be good regardless of the technique used provided the anastomosis into the nose is large.

The cut edges of the nasal and sac mucosas are sutured together with previously placed catgut sutures (Fig. 9-13). The deep tissues are carefully joined with about three interrupted sutures. Use of chromic catgut for this suturing may result in an inflammatory reaction with undue swelling, serious wound drainage, and unnecessary scarring. One of the sutures used to close the deep tissues may be passed through the sac and nasal mucosas to pull the mucosal flaps forward. Only if the sutured mucosal flaps tend to fall backward is this step indicated. Synthetic absorbable suture (5-0 or 6-0 Dexon, no. 7537-13, Davis & Geck Division, American Cyanamid Company) is satisfactory. The skin is sutured with 6-0 interrupted silk sutures; these can be removed 48 to 72 hours postoperatively.

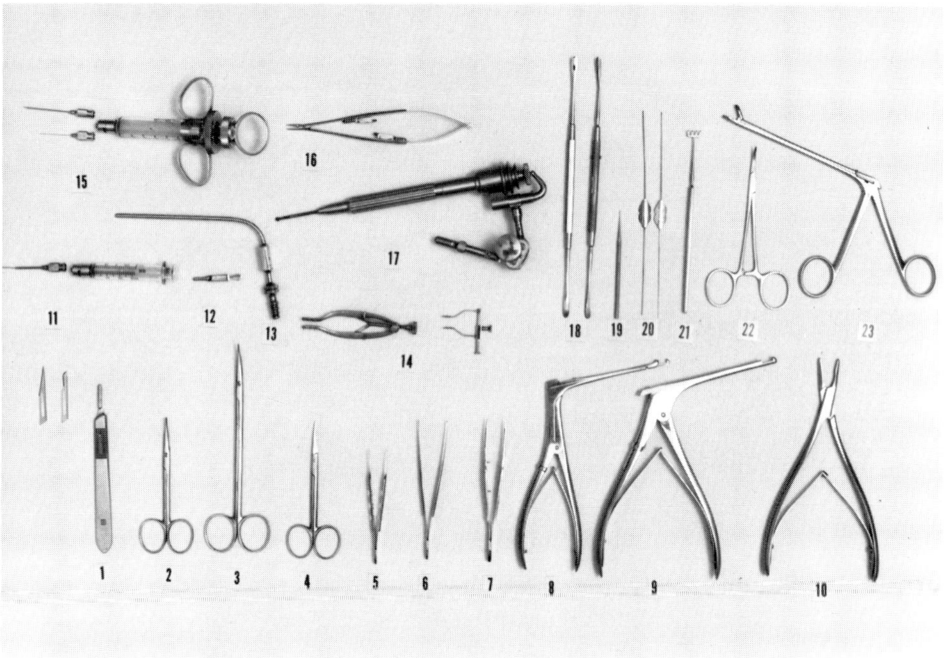

Fig. 9-14. Instruments used in routine external dacryocystorhinostomy. *1,* Bard-Parker knife handle with no. 11 and 15 blades; *2,* Stevens muscle scissors; *3,* Potts tenotomy scissors; *4,* suture scissors; *5,* Bishop Harmon forceps; *6,* large-tooth forceps; *7,* tying forceps; *8,* sphenoid punch forceps; *9,* Kerrison rongeur forceps; *10,* Lampert rongeur; *11,* 2-ml syringe with 23-gauge lacrimal needle; *12,* serrefine clamps; *13,* no. 3 suction tube; *14,* Stevenson and Goldstein lacrimal retractors; *15,* 5-ml syringe with 20- and 30-gauge needles; *16,* Castroviejo needle holder; *17,* Jordan Day drill with round cutting bur, 5/32-inch diameter; *18,* Freer elevators; *19,* punctum dilator; *20,* Bowman probes; *21,* rake retractors; *22,* Halsted mosquito forceps (curved); *23,* ethmoid punch.

Instruments

The instruments used for the procedure described above are shown in Fig. 9-14.

OTHER TECHNIQUES

In the method described by Dupuy-Dutemps and Bourget,[1] posterior flaps of lacrimal sac and nasal mucosa are fashioned and sutured together; anterior flaps also are sutured together. This technique can greatly increase the difficulty in suturing the mucosal flaps together, especially if the lacrimal sac is small or scarred or if the mucosa is damaged during the operation. If the sac and nasal mucosa available in a small, scarred, or damaged lacrimal sac is sufficient to allow both posterior and anterior flaps to be sutured, fashioning and suturing flaps as shown in Fig. 9-10 is far more satisfactory.

Except when operating on large lacrimal sacs, it is technically difficult to fashion posterior flaps and suture them together because of the small size and depth of the field. Incising part of the mucosa to use as posterior flaps may not leave sufficient mucosa for also fashioning anterior flaps that can be sutured to each other.

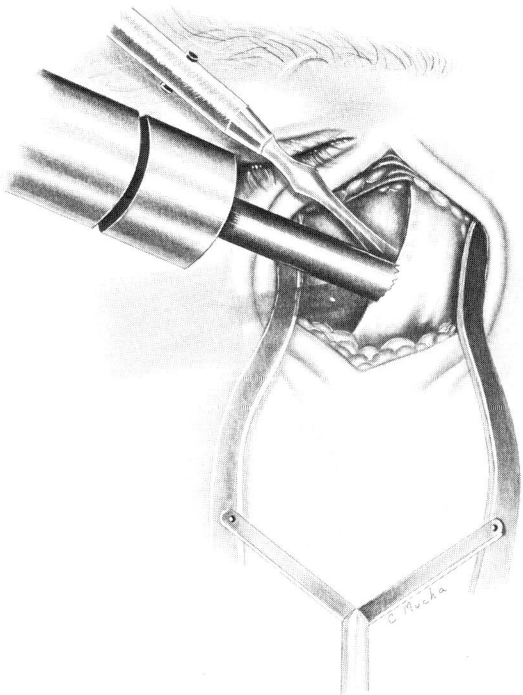

Fig. 9-15. Iliff method of removing bone with Stryker saw.

Kasper's[4] technique differs from most other techniques primarily in the method of handling the mucosal flaps. After sufficient bone is removed the exposed nasal mucosa is excised. Part of the middle turbinate is removed if it lies close to the osteotomy site. The sac mucosa is cut in a U shape by using a knife or scissors to make a continuous incision along the anterior, superior, and inferior edges of the sac. This flap, which in essence is the medial wall of the sac, is left hinged posteriorly and is then placed over the posterior margin of the osteotomy opening into the nose. No sutures are used in the flap.

Iliff[3] uses a Stryker saw with a special trephine to make the bony opening straddling the anterior lacrimal crest (Fig. 9-15). The diameter of the opening is 8 mm in children and 10 mm in adults. After the exposed nasal mucosa is incised or excised, one end of a 14-F urethral catheter cut to proper length is anchored by 3-0 chromic catgut in the neck of the sac. The other end of the catheter is anchored to the external nares. The catheter is left in position for 10 days.

TECHNIQUE FOR CASES WITH POOR PROGNOSIS

Many techniques have been advocated for improving the prognosis after an external dacryocystorhinostomy. The routine use of catheters, wicks, or other material extending through the newly formed anastomosis from the sac to the nose seems unwarranted. If the operation is properly performed, the outlook for cure is nearly 100% in favorable cases. When the outlook for cure is unfavorable, as in cases in which there is extensive scarring in and around the sac from previous operations or trauma, very small sacs, or tumor involving the sac, a special technique may be required to establish a permanent anastomosis.

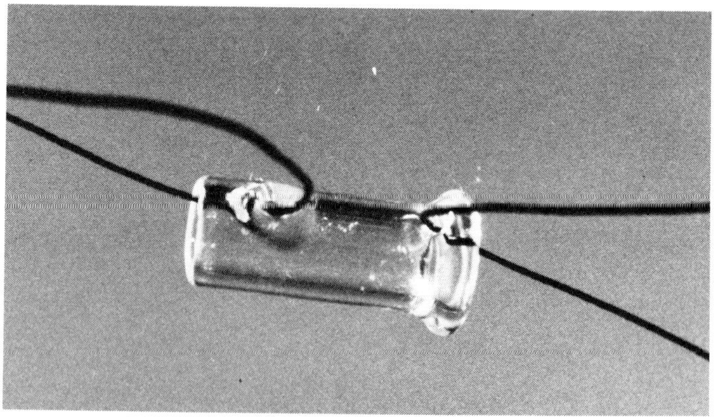

Fig. 9-16. Pyrex tube with perforation at both ends through which permanent sutures are threaded. Flanged end is sutured securely to soft tissues of inner wall of opened lacrimal sac so that tears can enter tube from canaliculus. Tube lies in newly formed anastomosis, the unflanged end emptying into nose.

In these cases the most satisfactory method is to insert a special Pyrex glass tube. The flanged end of this tube is sutured into position within the lacrimal sac with a permanent type of suture (Fig. 9-16). The unflanged end, which also has a perforation near its tip, extends into the nose. A permanent suture is passed through the perforation in the nasal tip of the Pyrex tube and tied, leaving about 2 cm or so loose (Fig. 9-17). If desired, this suture later may be grasped within the nose and used to pull the Pyrex tube out. As an additional hedge, the suture used to anchor the flanged end within the lacrimal sac may be cut sufficiently long to extend far enough into the nose to be grasped. The Pyrex tubes are constructed in different lengths, usually 5 to 8 mm in width at the flanged end and 4 to 6 mm at the unflanged end. (These tubes are made to order by Gunther Weiss, 2025 S. W. Briggs Court, Beaverton, Oregon.)

The tubes usually can be left in position permanently without irritation and with excellent results. If removal of the tube is indicated for any reason, the free ends of the permanent sutures that are tied to the tube can be grasped intranasally and the tube removed through the nares.

A

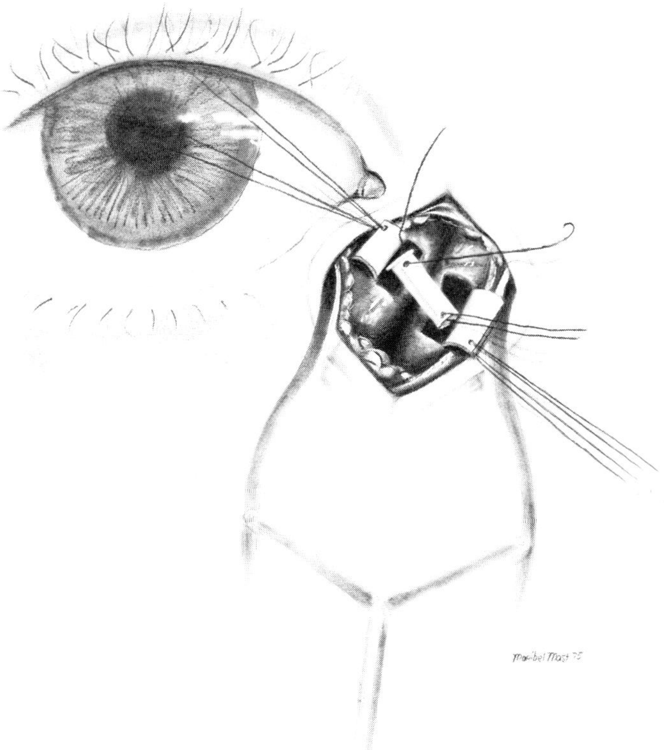

Continued.

Fig. 9-17. Placement of Pyrex tube. **A,** Mersilene 5-0 suture (Ethicon) is threaded through perforations in both ends of tube. Upper end of tube is carefully adjusted within sac, which is usually scarred and small. Lower end of tube extends into nose for 2 or 3 mm.

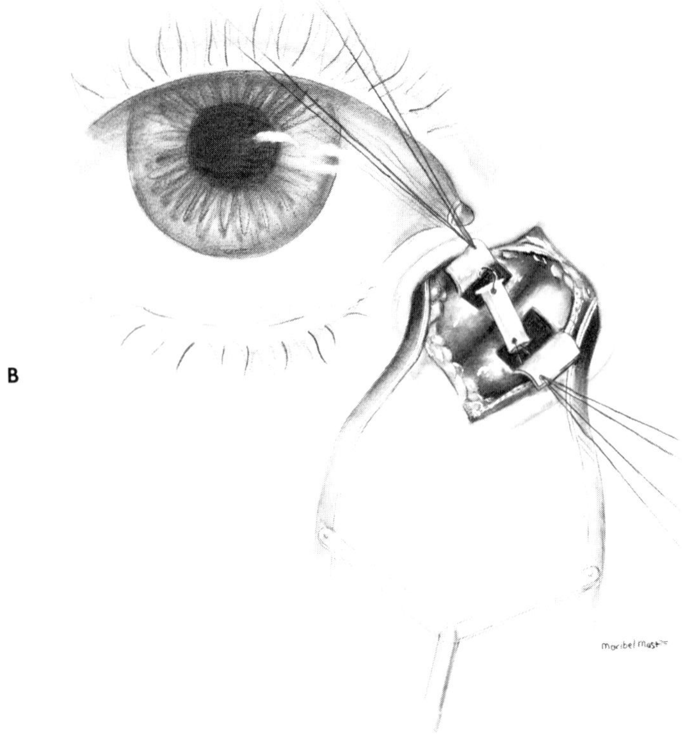

Fig. 9-17, cont'd. B, Upper end of tube is anchored securely by taking a substantial bite in sac tissues, and knot is tied in suture in lower perforation so it cannot be pulled loose from Pyrex tube. Lower suture is left about 2 cm long to pass into nose to pull Pyrex tube out if necessary. Lacrimal and mucosal flaps are sutured routinely.

POSTOPERATIVE CARE

A mild pressure dressing is applied to the side operated on. If bilateral dacryocystorhinostomies are performed at the same time, leaving one eye open seems to cause no problems. The patient should be warned preoperatively to expect some nasal bleeding, which varies from a minimal to an annoying amount. Elevation of the head of the bed for the first few hours postoperatively may help to lessen the oozing of blood. Most patients will require an analgesic on the day of operation, but few will thereafter. Patients are warned to avoid strenuous physical exercises, getting overheated, or forcefully blowing their nose. Hospitalization for 1 or 2 days is usually sufficient. Irrigation with isotonic saline through the canaliculi at the time of suture removal or a day or so later to remove possible obstructing material (blood clots, and so on) is advisable. Further postoperative care is seldom needed in routine cases.

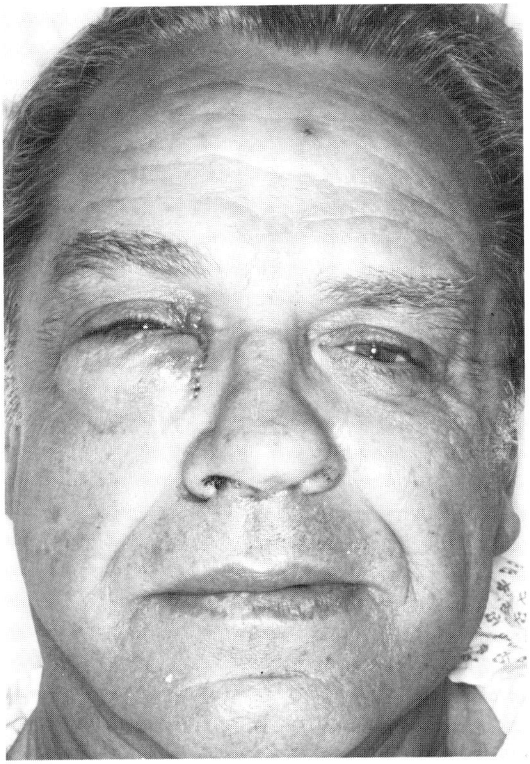

Fig. 9-18. Appearance of patient who blew his nose vigorously on day of operation, causing air to infiltrate soft tissues of lower lid.

COMPLICATIONS

Operative complications

Excessive bleeding. Patients should be cautioned not to engage in strenuous activities for 7 to 10 days postoperatively. Also, they are not to blow their nose forcefully (Fig. 9-18). Excessive bleeding, troublesome during the operation, is an annoyance but rarely is a serious complication. Insertion of the lacrimal speculum immediately after the soft tissue is incised usually will slow the bleeding. Clamping vessels with a hemostat and touching the hemostat with a cautery tip while the patient is grounded effectively stops the bleeding. Cautery can be applied freely to a bleeding nutrient vessel exiting from the exposed bone because this bone will later be removed. Minimal cautery may be applied to a bleeding vessel of the intact exposed mucosa.

Little bleeding is encountered when the lacrimal sac mucosa is incised. Bleeding may be profuse with the incision of the nasal mucosa, which should follow the fashioning of the lacrimal sac mucosa. Holding a pressure pack previously wetted with 1:10,000 epinephrine solution (with excess solution squeezed out) against the bleeding area may slow bleeding if the operation is performed under local anesthesia. If epinephrine is contraindicated, for example, in some instances when general anesthesia is used, 2.5% phenylephrine hydrochloride (Neo-Synephrine) may be substituted.

Excessive trauma to mucosa. The nasal or lacrimal sac mucosa may be torn inadvertently during the operation. If a drill is being used to remove the bone, the drill handle should be held with both hands, and one hand should be braced on the patient's face. This allows ample pressure to be applied to the drill for removing the bone without rupturing the nasal mucosa. Separating the mucosa from the bone with a periosteal elevator (Freer) will allow bone to be removed with biting forceps without damage to the mucosa.

If the nasal or sac mucosa is damaged, removal of sufficiently large amounts of bone will expose sufficient nasal mucosa to permit fashioning adequate mucosal flaps. Cauterizing the posterior and inferior lips of the wound with diathermy cautery will enlarge the anastomosis. If the sac is small or has been severely traumatized, placement of a specially constructed Pyrex tube from the sac into the nose may be needed.

Failure to identify lacrimal sac. Identification of the lacrimal sac should present no real difficulty in routine operations by experienced operators. The anterior lacrimal crest is the important landmark: the sac lies in its fossa laterally and posteriorly to the crest. The sac has a light grayish color. Passing a lacrimal probe through one of the canaliculi to tent the sac laterally is one way to identify it in case of doubt. It is possible to incise only the outer coat of the sac (the periosteum) without entering its lumen. The membrane lining of the lumen is usually easily recognizable. The lining has a light gray color; it may present either a smooth or a slightly papillary appearance. If the sac contains material such as mucopus or a dacryolith, identification is confirmed.

When there is some doubt, seeing the lacrimal probe that has been passed into the lacrimal sac through the canaliculus or injection of fluid or air into the sac through one of the canaliculi may be helpful. The most difficult lacrimal sacs to identify are the small ones, especially if surrounded by scar tissue from previous operations or injuries or if compressed by adjacent tissues such as a mucocele. When scar tissue is present, tenting the sac laterally with a lacrimal probe may not be possible. Careful dissection down to the inserted Bowman probe with Stevens scissors is the easiest and safest method to identify a lacrimal sac if the anatomy of the area has been altered by scarring or other pathologic processes.

Damage to canaliculus. Trauma to the entrance of the common canaliculus into the lacrimal sac may result in stenosis and continuing epiphora. Unhappily, this may occur despite the curing of the lacrimal sac infection. Unfortunately, stenosis of the ampullary portion of the common canaliculus may also be present preoperatively. Dacryocystography is the best method to detect this problem.

The medial palpebral tendon is the key landmark: the common canalicular opening is at this level. If the original incision is begun below the level of the medial palpebral tendon and other operative manipulations are also kept below this level, damage to the canaliculi from direct trauma to the common canalicular opening or torsion of the canaliculi due to faulty suturing is unlikely. In a few instances when there is an abnormality in the area of the common canalicular opening, the soft tissue incision may have to be extended superiorly to sever the medial palpebral tendon in order to expose the opening satisfactorily. If operative trauma to this area would seem likely to result in stenosis, insertion of a stainless steel canalicular rod is advisable.

Damage to contiguous structures. Orbital fat may extrude if the operative intervention is inadvertently carried through the periorbita that is lateral to the lacrimal sac. If this complication is recognized early, no damage results. The antrum may be entered when the bone is removed too far in the inferolateral direction. The lining membrane of the antrum is very thin in contrast to the lacrimal sac and nasal mucosa. No permanent damage results from entering the antrum if the opening is small.

Late complications

Postoperative bleeding. Hemorrhage of sufficient consequence to require special attention may occur on the day of operation or as late as 7 to 10 days postoperatively. If not too severe, simple measures such as keeping the patient in bed with the head elevated and ice packs applied to the operative area may suffice. A preoperative screen consisting of a prothrombin time, partial thromboplastin time, and platelet count may be of value in patients with a history of excessive bleeding or if there is abnormal postoperative bleeding. As a last resort, applying pressure to the bleeding area, the anastomosis, may be needed. This can be done by insertion of the pack into this area by an otolaryngologist if necessary.

Closure of anastomosis. A thorough examination should be carried out. This includes examination of the nose, lids, puncta, and canaliculi, irrigation, and most importantly, dacryocystography. If the lacrimal sac can be demonstrated but the anastomosis is closed, reoperation usually is indicated. A repeat external dacryocystorhinostomy with special modification will yield the highest percentage of good results. This is especially true if the lacrimal sac is at least of moderate size or larger. In many instances the previously made anastomosis from the sac into the nose was too small. In more difficult situations, such as when there is dense scarring or a very small lacrimal sac, insertion of a small Pyrex tube at reoperation is indicated (see p. 130).

In a few instances a Bowman probe can be passed through the upper or lower canaliculus and an opening forced into the nose at the site of the closed anastomosis. A hemostat is used to grasp the nasal end of the Bowman probe within the nose while the punctal end is held by the other hand. The anastomosis may

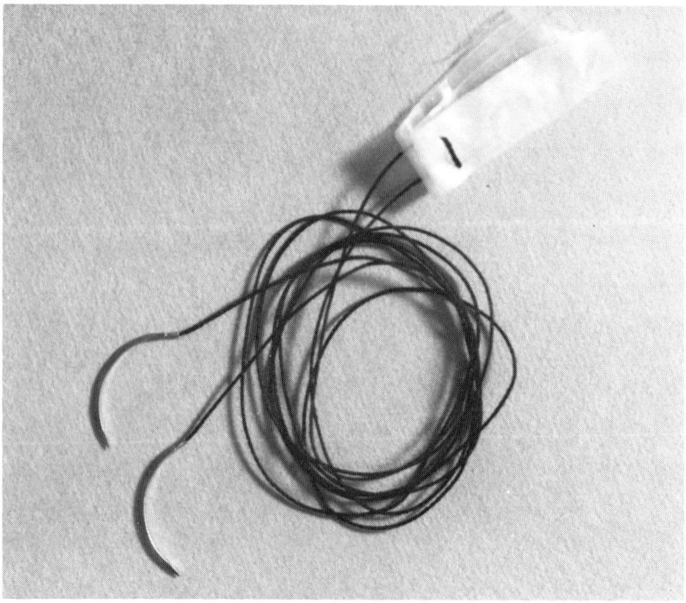

Fig. 9-19. A 5-0 suture passed through strips of folded polyethylene sheeting. Needle is cut off, and knot is tied to secure strips together.

be enlarged by vigorously forcing the probe held at both its ends in anteroposterior, lateral, and circular directions.

If the operator is sufficiently adept, a 5-0 Vicryl double-arm (Ethicon) suture can be attached to the nasal end of the probe through a perforation in one end of the probe and drawn upward through the anastomosis and upper canaliculus; thus, the suture will extend from the external nares upward and out the upper punctum. The lower end of this suture is passed through folded strips of polyethylene sheeting 4 to 6 mm in length (Fig. 9-19), and the strips are pulled into the freshly "reamed out" anastomosis by pulling upward on the suture that exits from the upper punctum. A free needle is threaded onto this end of the suture, a bite is taken in the soft tissue adjacent to the punctum, and a knot is tied to hold the sheeting in the anastomosis. Excess length of the nasal end of the suture is cut. The sheeting is removed after 6 to 8 weeks. This procedure does not carry as favorable a prognosis as repeated dacryocystorhinostomy, but if properly performed in cases in which the anastomosis is not securely closed, a permanent opening can be established.

Unsightly scarring. Every effort should be made to avoid ugly scars. Most are avoidable. In making the incision through the skin and other soft tissues, the thumb of the left hand should be pressed firmly against the patient's nose just above the medial palpebral tendon. This allows the operator better control as the incision is swept downward. The blade of the knife should be kept at a right angle to the skin to avoid a slanting incision into the soft tissues.

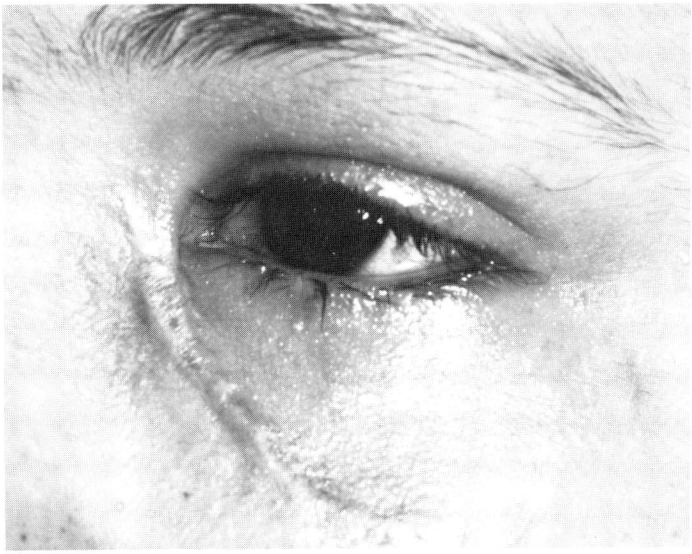

Fig. 9-20. Severe bowstring scar as result of overly curved incision extended too far superiorly. (From Veirs, E.: Summary. In Veirs, E., editor: The lacrimal system: Proceedings of the first international symposium, St. Louis, 1970, The C. V. Mosby Co., pp. 157-173.)

The incision is started just inferiorly and 3 to 5 mm laterally to the inner canthus and is carried boldly downward for 20 to 25 mm. It should include all of the soft tissues down through the periosteum. If the incision is directed straight downward, usually the operator will discover that the incision is curved nearly parallel to the anterior lacrimal crest, an ideal incision. If the operator intentionally curves the incision laterally to any degree, the curve obtained is much greater than desired. Unsightly bowstring scars may result (Fig. 9-20).

To avoid a depression at the site of the skin incision, the muscle and other deep tissues should be carefully sutured after suturing of the mucosal flap (Fig. 9-21). If scar formation seems to be excessive, an injection of a long-acting steroid suspension such as triamcinolone acetonide (Kenalog-10 injection) into the scar is recommended; a repeat injection may be given in 2 to 3 weeks to help minimize the scarring.

Persistent edema. Persistent edema is annoying and if of sufficient severity may subside only slowly (Fig. 9-22). It requires no treatment.

Persistent epiphora. Epiphora persisting after a satisfactory external dacryocystorhinostomy may be due to (1) unrecognized stenosis of the canaliculi, most commonly a partial stenosis of the common canaliculus, (2) disorders of the eyelids such as a weakness of the orbicularis oculi muscles from paresis or from loss of tonicity as a result of age or injury, or (3) atrophy of the lacrimal sac, a possible but perhaps not plausible cause.

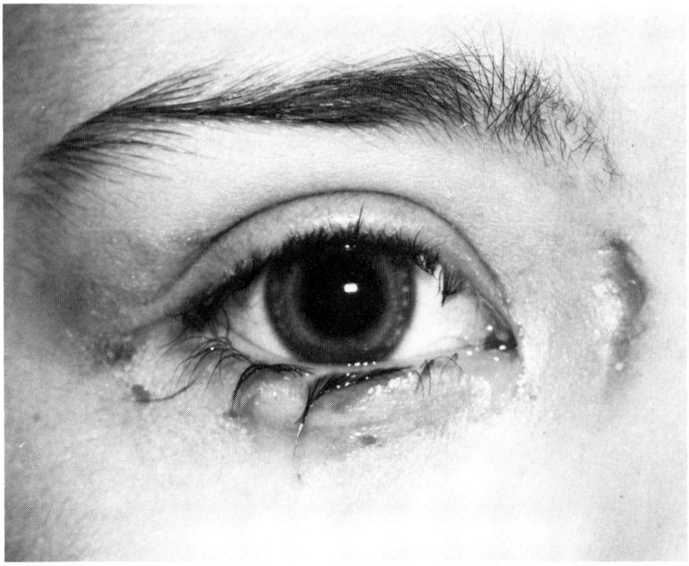

Fig. 9-21. Depressed scar resulted when incision was made too high and wound was not adequately sutured.

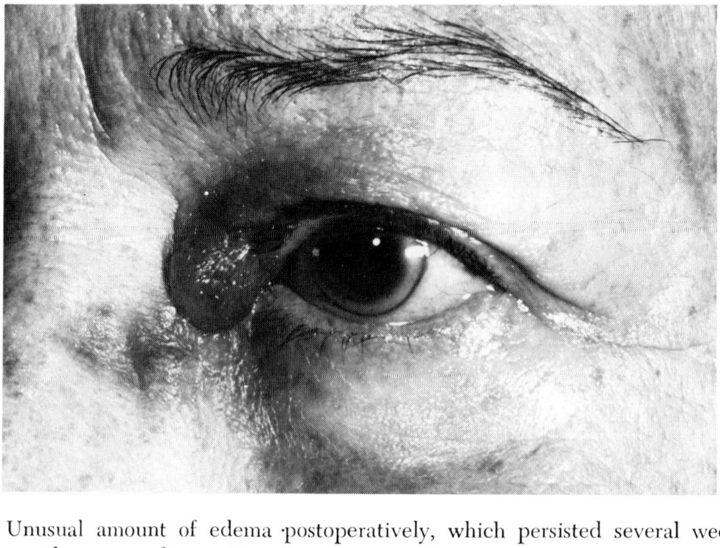

Fig. 9-22. Unusual amount of edema postoperatively, which persisted several weeks. It did not interfere with success of operation.

Blowing air into the eye. This is not a true complication. Patients may be alarmed that air blows into the eye when they blow their nose. They only need to be reassured that this is a sure sign that the anastomosis is patent. Mentioning that this may happen postoperatively prepares the patient for the event.

Infection. Serious postoperative infections are rare, and antibiotics usually are not indicated. An annoying stitch abscess occurs occasionally.

SUMMARY

External dacryocystorhinostomy offers a high percentage of permanent cures (about 95%) of dacryocystitis when the operation is properly executed in routine cases. Results are most likely to be satisfactory when (1) the operator has a thorough understanding of the anatomy and physiology of the lacrimal drainage system; (2) the operator has had adequate training including some experience with intranasal manipulations; (3) the patient has had a thorough preoperative workup including an accurate history, examination, and inspection of the lids, puncta, canaliculi, lacrimal sac, and nasolacrimal duct (dacryocystography is especially helpful); and (4) experienced assistants and good operative equipment are available.

The routine insertion of wicks, catheters, or other devices at the time of a primary external dacryocystorhinostomy seldom enhances the chances of success. Their use should be limited to the few cases in which closure of the anastomosis might otherwise be expected. Making a large anastomosis from the lacrimal sac into the nose in the proper position is far and away the most important measure to ensure success. Fashioning and suturing mucosal flaps, cauterizing the posterior and inferior lips of the anastomosis, and other measures undoubtedly improve the success rate but to a lesser degree. Finally, removal of the lacrimal sac as a substitute for dacryocystorhinostomy is to be strongly condemned. Malignancy of the lacrimal sac is the only indication for dacryocystectomy.

REFERENCES

1. Dupuy-Dutemps, and Bourget: Cure de la dacryocystite chronique et du larmoiement par la dacryorhinostomie plastique, Presse med, Par 30:833-835, 1922.
2. Hecht, S. D.: Internal common punctum during dacryocystorhinostomy. Accurate localization by the irrigation and bubble technique, Arch Ophthalmol 89:124, 1973.
3. Iliff, C. E.: A simplified dacryocystorhinostomy: 1954 to 1970, Trans Am Acad Ophthalmol Otolaryngol 75:821-828, 1971.
4. Kasper, K. A.: Dacryocystorhinostomy, Sur Ophthalmol 6:95-107, 1961.
5. Picó, G.: A modified technique of external dacryocystorhinostomy, Am J Ophthalmol 72: 679-690, 1971.
6. Toti, A.: Nuovo metodo conservatore di cura radicale delle suppurazioni croniche del sacco lacrimale (dacriocistorinostomia), Clin Med 10:385, 1904.

CHAPTER 10

Reconstructive surgery

FRESHLY SEVERED CANALICULI

Freshly severed canaliculi are not common. They are seen more often in city hospitals that have a large trauma service. Many such cases, especially in adults, are readily recognizable; others, especially in the young, may be easily overlooked. If the patient is cooperative, isotonic saline is injected through the punctum of the involved lid. If the canaliculus is torn, the saline will exit at that point. In instances of doubt in the young a general anesthetic should be given to permit careful determination of the extent of the injury and to prepare the patient for whatever repair is needed.

If the ophthalmologist does not feel confident in his ability to repair fresh injuries to the inner canthal region, especially if injury to the canaliculi is suspected, the patient should be referred to one who is experienced in this type of work.

Etiology. Countless types of injuries may damage the canaliculi. In young children, dog bite is one of the most common causes of injury to either the upper or the lower canaliculus or both canaliculi—without injury to other adjacent structures, in my experience.

Contusion injuries (such as from falling against an object), getting the lid caught in wire, and industrial accidents of many types may damage the canaliculus (Fig. 10-1).

Diagnosis. This may be simple when the canaliculus is severed near the punctum by a knifelike vertical cut without injury to contiguous structures. Other injuries to the canaliculus may be much more subtle, and an involved lid displaced laterally a few millimeters may be the only external sign. The diagnosis may be difficult to prove if the inner canthal region is severely macerated or if the canaliculus is injured on a slant or medially near the common canaliculus. Few injuries are so severe that patency cannot be reestablished in most cases (Fig. 10-2).

If the injured tissues are greatly swollen and bleeding, a delay of 24 to 48 hours will allow the edema to subside and the bleeding to stop. With a clear field, the cut ends of the canaliculus stand out like pearly rings and are easily

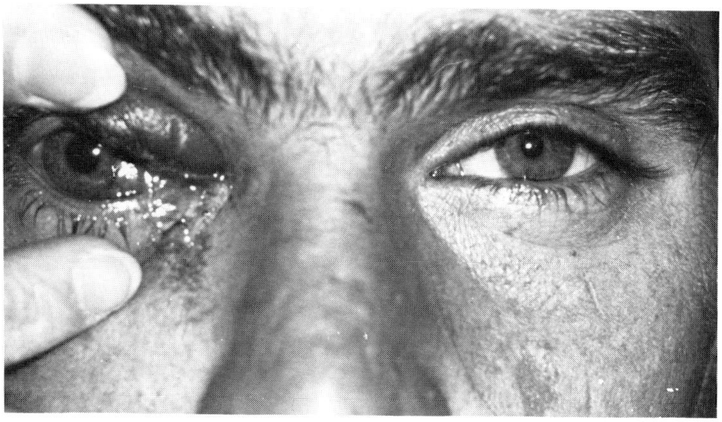

Fig. 10-1. Upper and lower canaliculi severed as result of industrial accident. Medial rectus muscle was sheared off at its insertion.

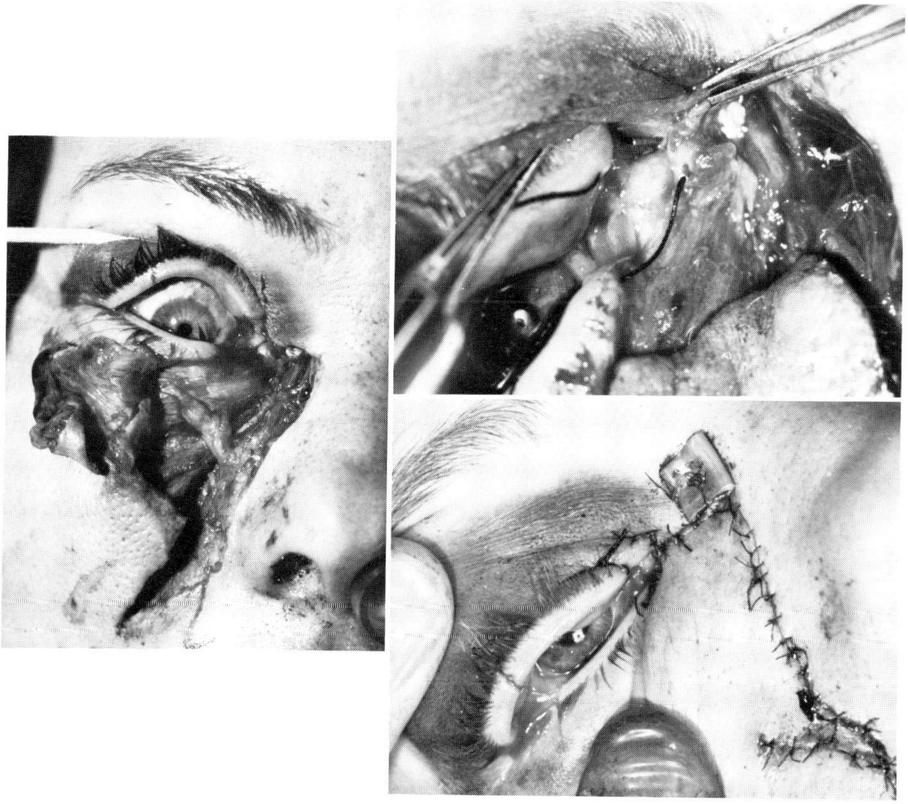

A

B

C

Fig. 10-2. Patient with facial injuries incurred from fall in bathroom. **A,** Preoperative appearance; both canaliculi were severed. **B,** Canalicular rods have been passed through both puncta and into medial cut ends of canaliculi. **C,** Cut edges of canaliculi have been carefully approximated by suture. Canalicular rods bridge severed canaliculi and lie entirely within canaliculi so that only the swaged 4-0 silk suture is exiting from puncta. This suture is secured in position by taking bite in soft tissues near puncta.

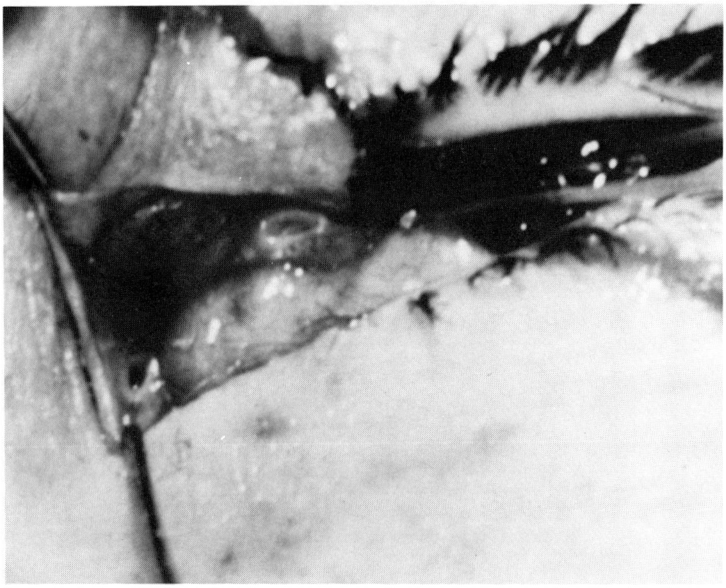

Fig. 10-3. Appearance of severed canaliculus 48 hours after injury. Bleeding and edema have subsided; severed ends are easily recognizable.

recognized (Fig. 10-3). Thus, a short delay may make repair much more satisfactory. If repair is to be delayed for 24 to 48 hours, the wound can be thoroughly lavaged when the patient is first examined. A delay of 48 hours does not seem to lessen the chances of successful repair. When the repair is properly performed, success can be achieved with a delay of as long as 5 days, but delaying this long is not desirable.

When only one canaliculus is involved, air is an excellent aid in localizing the proximal severed end. In the technique described by Morrison[2] a tampon is inserted under the anterior end of the inferior meatus to close the nasal end of the nasolacrimal duct. I have not found this necessary because when the patient is lying supine with face upward, the isotonic saline will stay in the wound. If the lower canaliculus is severed, a few milliliters of isotonic saline is injected through the intact upper canaliculus on the same side. Sufficient saline will collect in the wound, or 2 ml or so of saline also can be put directly into the wound. A lacrimal cannula is attached to a small syringe (2- or 5-ml) filled with air. As air is forced into the upper canaliculus, the bubbles can be seen exiting through the proximal severed end of the lower canaliculus.

Repair. The fact that countless techniques and modifications of techniques have been advocated for repair of freshly severed canaliculi is an indication that results are often not favorable.

Various suture materials, including catgut, silk, nylon, and Dacron, have been used for intubation of injured canaliculi. Plastic tubing, especially polyethylene and silicone, is commonly threaded into the injured canaliculus to bridge the severed ends prior to suturing of the wound. The tubing is anchored in position by many methods.

Worst[6] designed a pigtail probe for locating the medial severed end of the canaliculus as well as for pulling the tubing into position. This probe has been modified by others. Many ophthalmologists find it difficult to use, and some believe that damage to the canaliculus occurs because it has to be inserted blindly.

In my method a specifically designed[5] stainless steel rod, 12 mm long and 0.61 mm in diameter, is used (available as Eye-703G canalicular rod, Ethicon, Inc., Somerville, N.J.). A 4-0 black braided silk suture is swaged to one end; the other end is slightly tapered.

All freshly severed canaliculi, upper and lower if both are involved, should be repaired unless the procedure is contraindicated because of age or poor health of the patient. It is true that a single patent canaliculus may drain tears fairly well in some patients, especially those not exposed to external irritation such as cold windy weather or fumes. However, if both canaliculi are severed, but only one is repaired, or if a single severed canaliculus is not repaired, there is no protection against the consequences of subsequent stenosis of the single patent canaliculus on that side. The reason for the poor prognosis is improper repair. Many ophthalmologists have difficulty in achieving patency.

This procedure can be performed satisfactorily under local anesthesia in patients who have suffered a sharp cut through the canaliculus at a site not too far medially. When the injury is more severe and tissues are macerated or the lid avulsed (Fig. 10-4) or when it occurs in the young, general anesthesia is needed. Identification of the proximal (medial) severed end of the cut canaliculus is confirmed if isotonic saline instilled into it can be detected flowing into the nose.

The free end of a stainless steel canalicular rod is passed through the punctum of the severed canaliculus and into the medial portion of it. The stainless steel rod is placed entirely within the injured canaliculus to bridge the cut. The 4-0 silk suture that is swaged to the canalicular rod exits from the punctum (Fig. 10-5). The continuity of the injured canaliculus should be reestablished by carefully suturing—if possible, in the same way that an artery is sutured end to end. The first suture layer joins the two cut ends of the canaliculus (Fig. 10-6). Poor suturing of the wound may result not only in failure to reestablish a patent canaliculus but also in a cosmetically unacceptable result.

The buried suture material should have great tensile strength, be small in diameter, have a small half-curved needle, and be double-armed. If absorbable, the suture should have an effective holding time of about 3 weeks. Acceptable materials are 7-0 Vicryl (manufactured by Ethicon Inc., Somerville, N.J.) and 7-0 silk used as double-armed sutures to bring the cut edges of the canaliculus together. Then, 5-0 Vicryl or a suture of a similar strength may be used to repair a badly lacerated canaliculus that tends to pull laterally (Fig. 10-7).

The tissue holding the severed ends of the canaliculus should be sutured in

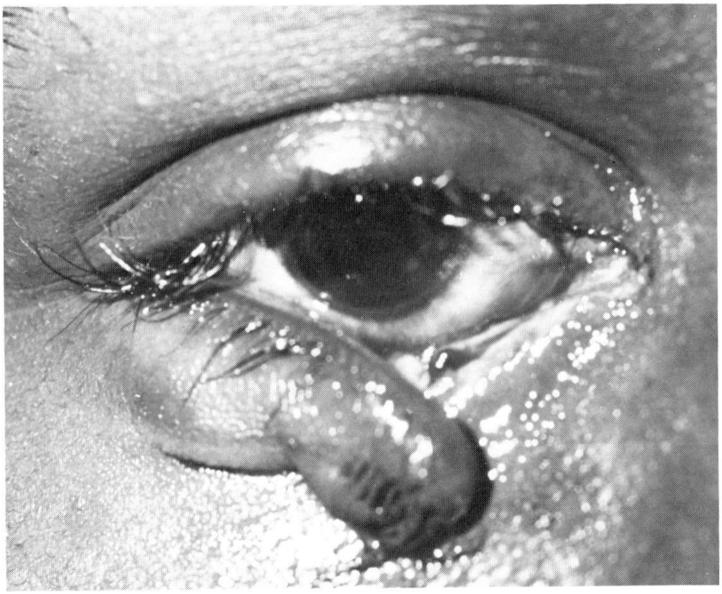

Fig. 10-4. Injury by hook resulted in torn lid and severed canaliculus. In repair of lower lid, suture of high tensile strength was used to prevent torn lid from pulling laterally.

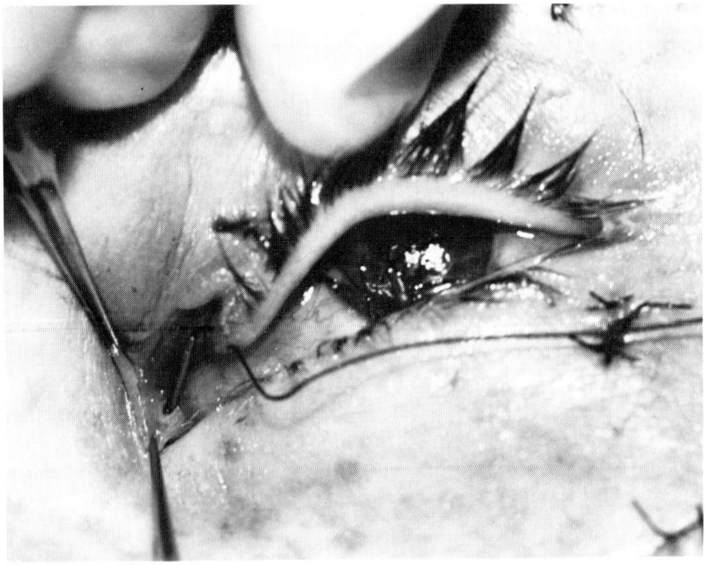

Fig. 10-5. Temporal end of canalicular rod has been passed into upper punctum; medial end has been inserted into proximal cut end of canaliculus. Note 4-0 silk suture, swaged on end of rod, emerging from punctum.

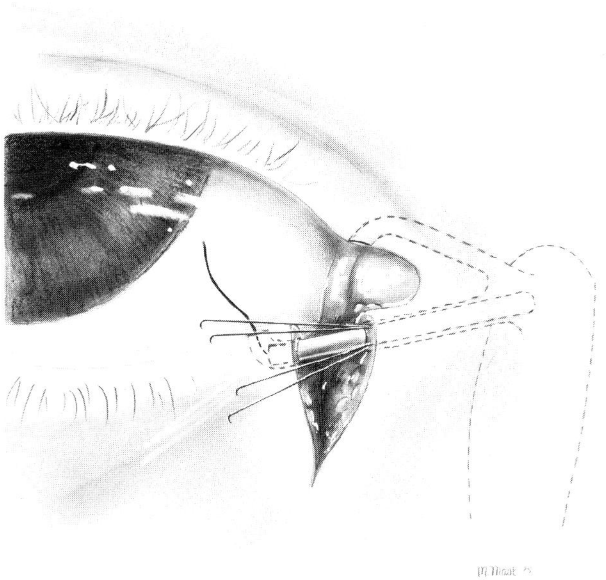

Fig. 10-6. Schematic representation of repair of severed canaliculus. A 12-mm-long canalicular rod has been passed through punctum to bridge severed canaliculus and enter medial cut end of canaliculus; 4-0 silk suture swaged to end of rod exits from punctum. Two fine double-armed sutures have been placed close to severed canaliculus medially and are ready to be sutured similarly to lateral portion of severed canaliculus. Second layer of sutures is then placed.

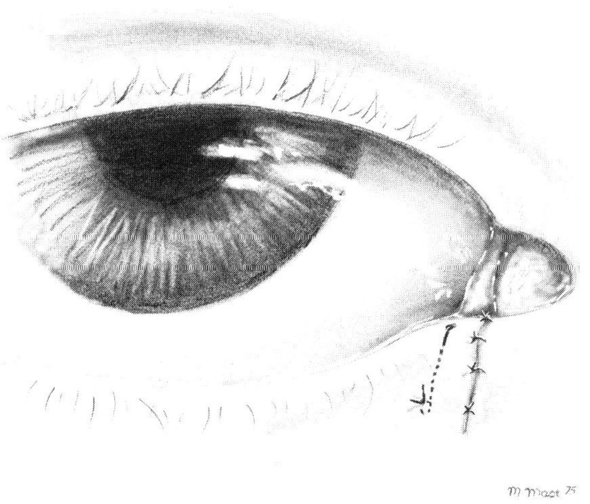

Fig. 10-7. Two layers of previously placed (buried) sutures have been tied, bringing incised edges of lid together and approximating cut edges of canaliculus. Skin sutures are carefully placed. With needle threaded onto 4-0 silk that exits from punctum, this suture is passed beneath skin for 10 mm and knotted securely after it exits from the skin.

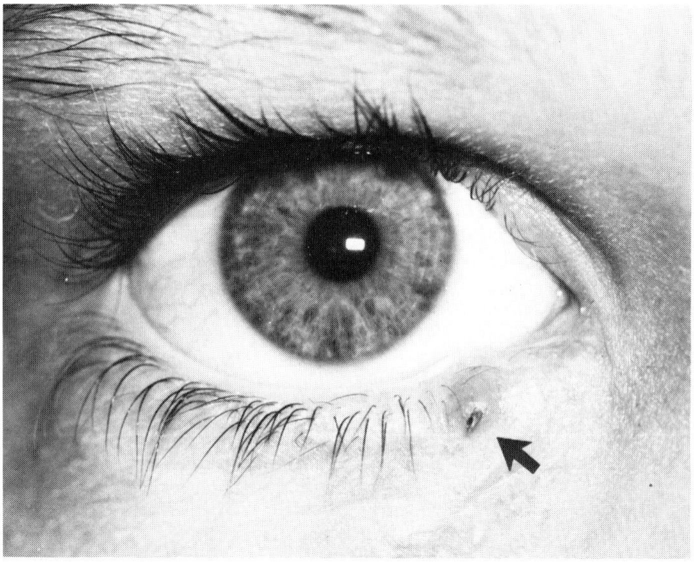

Fig. 10-8. After repair of severed canaliculus, child rubbed knot where it exited from skin, causing irritation. Knot was cut, leaving 4-0 silk *(arrow)* to be grasped for removal of canalicular rod at appropriate time.

several layers. Double-armed sutures seem to be preferable for most of the suturing. After the canaliculus has been sutured, a needle is threaded onto the free end of the 4-0 silk that is swaged on the canalicular rod and is exiting through the punctum. A vertically dissected bite is taken in the skin adjacent to the punctum and carried subcutaneously for 3 or 4 mm vertically where the needle and suture are brought to the surface. Another bite is taken in the soft tissue within a millimeter or so, a knot is tied securely, and the excess 4-0 silk is cut away. The canalicular rod is left in position for 6 to 12 weeks, depending on the severity of the injury.

The patient should be warned to keep the involved inner canthal region clean and not to rub the 4-0 silk knot. In the very young such warning may be to no avail. The knot rarely becomes untied, but if it does, part of the excess suture should be cut off and the rod left in place (Fig. 10-8). If the lid is severely torn or avulsed, anchoring the lid medially in its proper position requires sutures with adequate strength, and the sutures must be securely placed. Otherwise, the torn medial portion of the lid will pull laterally. In badly damaged lids, performing a tarsorrhaphy just lateral to the puncta may prevent development of ectropion. The tarsorrhaphy should not be performed until the canaliculus is repaired, including anchoring the rod in place.

Use of the stainless steel canalicular rod has the following advantages: (1) ease in placement (compared with the use of tubes, sutures, or other materials); (2) prevention of kinking that could interfere with healing (by splinting the

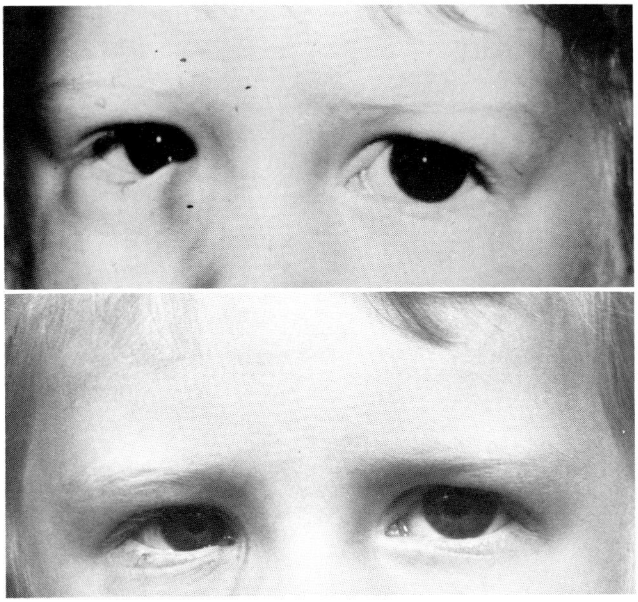

Fig. 10-9. Patient with congenital occlusion of lacrimal puncta on right with marked constant swelling of lacrimal sac but no evidence of inflammation. *Top,* Preoperative appearance. *Bottom,* Appearance 1 year postoperatively. Condition was corrected by using lacrimal sac mucosa to line part of newly created channel from lacrimal lake region (see text). No epiphora or swelling since operation.

repaired severed canaliculus); (3) avoidance of damage to the punctum or slitting of the canaliculus; (4) almost total absence of irritation (except for a rare stitch abscess, in which case the 4-0 silk knot is untied, and the silk is cut within 2 mm or so of the skin, leaving the rod in place as long as desired); (5) virtual impossibility of rod migration; (6) patient comfort; (7) high percentage of cures; and (8) elimination of danger of damaging the uninvolved canaliculus by use of a pigtail probe.

TOTAL RECONSTRUCTION OF LACRIMAL DRAINAGE SYSTEM

Total obstruction of the drainage of tears from the conjunctival sac into the nose occurs as the result of many pathologic processes. Establishment of a normal flow of tears may be extremely simple and permanent, for example, when congenital obstruction of the lacrimal ducts in infants is opened by probing. The routine external dacryocystorhinostomy is nearly 100% successful and requires only a few days of attention if all goes as expected.

Any reconstruction of the drainage system that requires bypassing stenosed canaliculi or correction for a lacrimal sac that for all practical purposes is absent involves surgical procedures that can be difficult to perform and an experience that is trying for the patient. Great patience over an extended time may be required from the ophthalmologist and the patient. Yet, many of these patients will get excellent functional results without much postoperative care (Fig. 10-9).

A good general rule is to avoid these procedures if there is a reasonable chance that an alternate approach will nearly duplicate the normal drainage system. For example, if the canaliculus opens into only a nubbin of a lacrimal sac, connecting this small pouch of a sac to the nose will usually provide satisfactory function even though the sac may have been severely damaged from injury or operations.

Indications for total reconstruction

The prime prerequisite for total reconstruction is the qualification of the surgeon. He should have the ability to perform a thorough examination and to identify accurately the cause of the epiphora. Unfortunately, lacrimal surgery is all but ignored by many training programs. The ophthalmologist must learn to use a head mirror, familiarize himself thoroughly with that part of the nose to be operated on, and become reasonably adept at using the instruments needed. The operator should be endowed with ample patience and ideally should choose patients who live close by.

Patients with epiphora that is causing considerable annoyance and that cannot be corrected by easier means should be considered as candidates for some type of reconstructive surgery. The most common causes are (1) congenital absence of the canaliculi, the lacrimal sac, or both, (2) stenosis of the canaliculi that is too extensive to repair, and (3) absence of the lacrimal sac as a result of injury or disease.

Operative techniques

Once the patient has undergone a thorough examination of the drainage system and the decision has been made that the symptoms warrant some type of reconstructive surgery, the decision is made as to what type of reconstructive surgery is indicated. Any intranasal pathologic process that might interfere with success is corrected prior to the lacrimal surgery.

Use of lacrimal sac mucosa alone. A rare condition is congenital absence of the canaliculi and occlusion of the nasolacrimal duct. I have seen two patients with bilateral involvement and one with unilateral involvement. The lacrimal sacs were enormously enlarged and filled with mucoid secretion but not infected. All three patients were between 7 and 10 years old; the swelling had been present since birth.

An incision is made similar to that of an external dacryocystorhinostomy except that the original incision (vertical) is made about 4 mm or more nasally to the inner canthus to avoid incising into the lacrimal sac. The bone separating the sac from the nasal mucosa is removed as for an external dacryocystorhinostomy, and the removal is extended as far inferiorly as practical.

A vertical rectangular flap of lacrimal sac mucosa is cut in the anteromedial

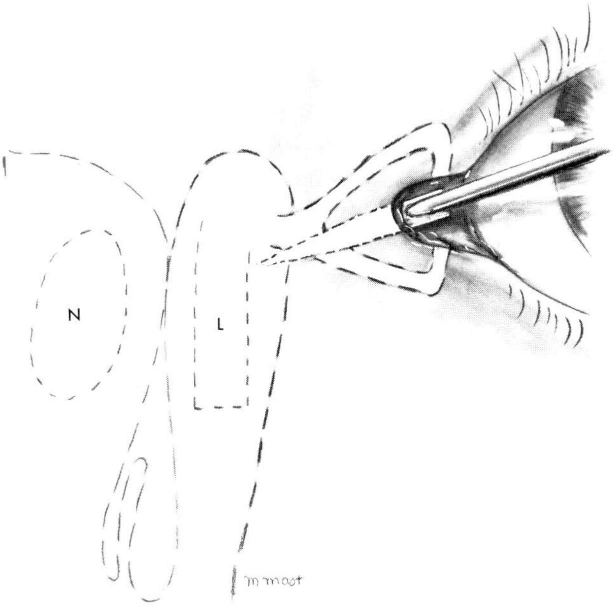

Fig. 10-10. Rectangular flap, *L*, is fashioned from lacrimal sac mucosa. Oval portion, *N*, of nasal mucosa is cut away. Caruncle has been removed, and sharp-pointed knife is used to make channel from lacus lacrimalis through soft tissues into lacrimal sac. Channel is enlarged with small curved hemostat.

aspect of the sac (Fig. 10-10) so that its lower end can be swung upward, brought out the lacus lacrimalis (previously prepared by removal of the caruncle, thus creating a channel from the lacus lacrimalis to the lacrimal sac), and sutured to the conjunctiva (Fig. 10-11). Approximately half the circumference of this new channel is thus lined with sac mucosa, and the other half is unlined; its length is about 5 mm.

A Pyrex tube (Fig. 10-12) about 6 mm long, 3 mm in diameter at its nasal end, and with a small hole in its eye (flanged) end is inserted into the newly formed channel. The tube is anchored into position by passing a Dacron suture through the hole in the flanged end of the tube and into tissue in the lacus lacrimalis. The tube is left in position for 3 to 4 months (longer if necessary) until the raw surface of the channel epithelializes. The nasal mucosa opposing the lacrimal sac is removed to provide a large opening into the nose. The cut edges of the nasal mucosa are cauterized to prevent closure.

Use of nasal mucosa. A somewhat similar operation utilizes a similarly shaped flap of nasal mucosa. An external dacryocystorhinostomy is performed. To ensure that sufficient nasal mucosa is available for the flap, the bone is removed as far inferiorly and superiorly as is practical. It is especially important to remove as much bone superiorly as is safe. This not only allows a longer rectangle of

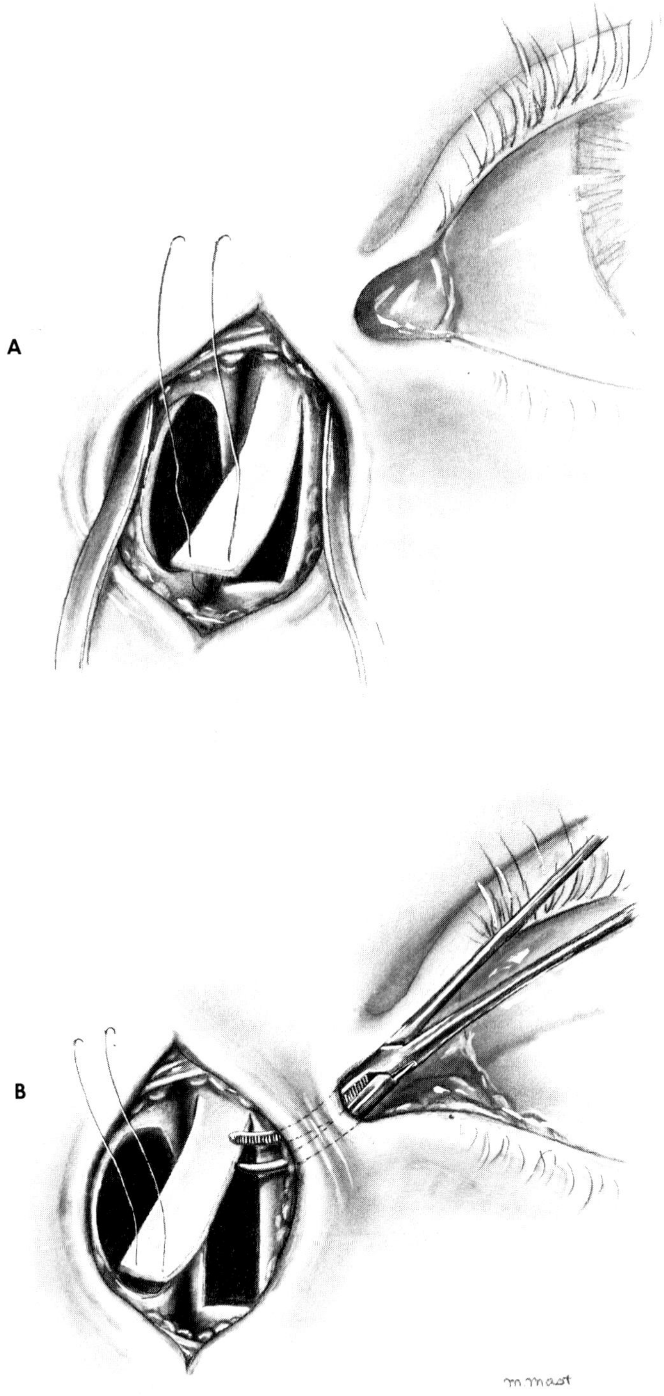

Fig. 10-11. A, Double-armed sutures placed through lower end of flap of lacrimal sac mucosa. **B,** Curved hemostat is passed through newly formed channel from lacus lacrimalis into lacrimal sac area to grasp needle ends of previously placed suture. **C,** Flap of lacrimal sac mucosa is drawn through newly created channel. Care is exercised that raw surface of this flap will lie flat on one side of new channel. **D,** Flap of lacrimal mucosa is sutured to conjunctiva, with raw surface posteriorly.

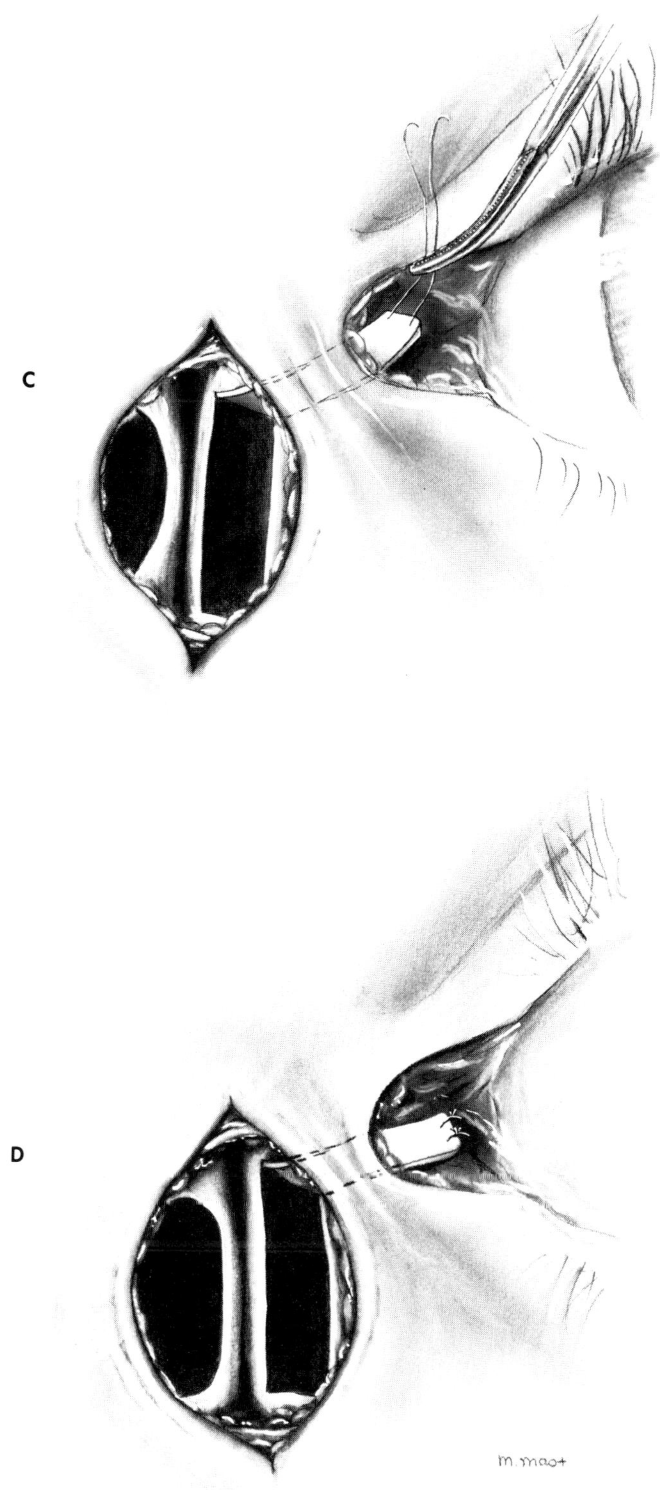

Fig. 10-11, cont'd. For legend see opposite page.

A

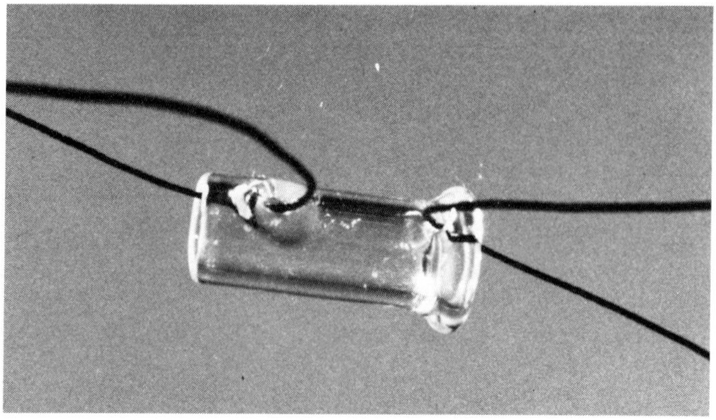

B

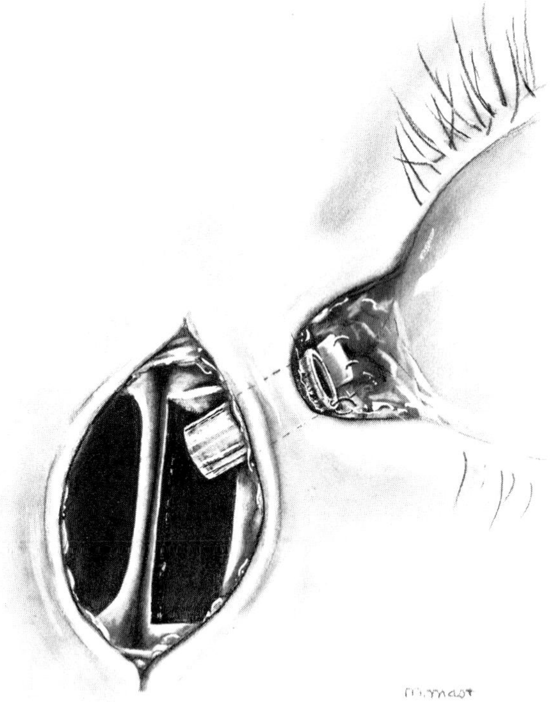

Fig. 10-12. A, Small Pyrex tube to be inserted into newly created channel to lie anterior to lacrimal sac mucosa. **B,** Flanged end lies in lacus lacrimalis and is anchored in position by threading a needle on free end of suture and taking a bite in adjacent soft tissues. Suture is not needed on unflanged end, which will lie in lacrimal sac region.

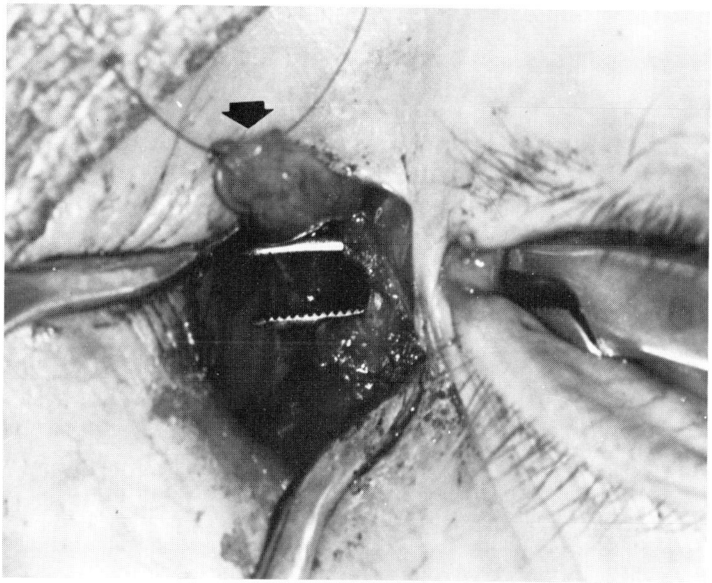

Fig. 10-13. Bone separating lacrimal sac from nasal mucosa has been removed. Rectangular flap *(arrow)* of nasal mucosa was fashioned to hinge superiorly, and mattress suture was placed. Curved hemostat is enlarging channel created from lacus lacrimalis to large opening into nose. Hemostat will grasp suture to pull flap of nasal mucosa laterally to be sutured to conjunctiva.

nasal mucosal flap (hinged superiorly) to be fashioned but also produces a shorter channel for the flap to line. (The flap does not have to bend around bone superiorly.) A double-armed suture is placed through the tongue of nasal mucosa near its tip, which lies inferiorly until swung upward as shown in Fig. 10-11, *upper left*. If the nasal mucosa flap is unduly thick (the mucosa is thicker inferiorly), it can easily be thinned prior to insertion of the mattress sutures.

The caruncle is excised, and a new channel is produced by passing a no. 11 Bard-Parker blade or other sharp instrument nasally from the area where the caruncle was removed to the large nasal opening as shown in Fig. 10-10. This new channel can be enlarged by manipulation of a curved hemostat (Fig. 10-13). The double-armed suture previously placed through the nasal mucosal flap is grasped with the hemostat and pulled through the new channel into the lacrimal lake region and sutured to the conjunctiva. It is of utmost importance for the raw surface of the tongue of nasal mucosa to lie on the raw surface of the new channel.

The Pyrex tube that is then inserted must lie on the epithelial surface of the nasal mucosal flap (Fig. 10-14). This tube is anchored into position by passing a Dacron suture through the perforation in its flanged end.

Comment. A patent channel can be similarly constructed by using a nasal mucosal flap as described and a flap of bulbar conjunctivae sutured to each other.[3]

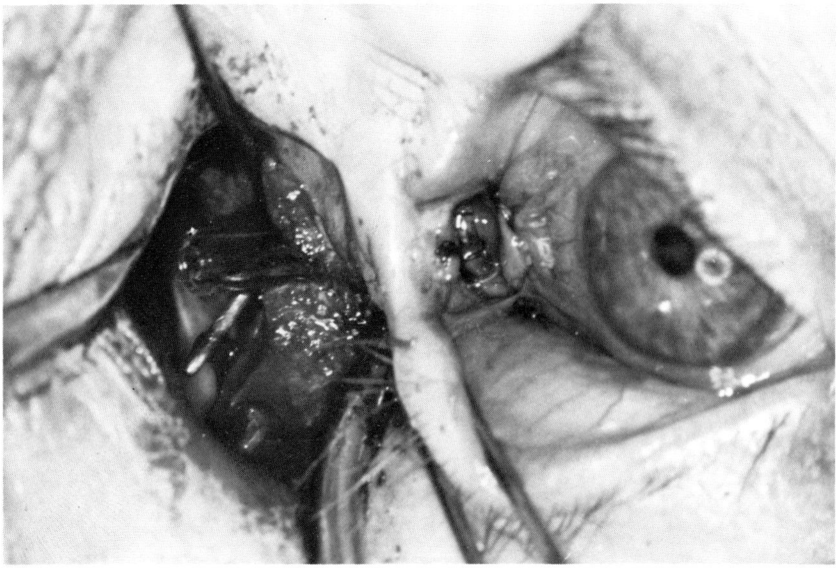

Fig. 10-14. Pyrex tube has been inserted and anchored in position with Dacron suture passed through small hole at flanged end. Tip of nasal mucosa flap can be seen sutured to conjunctiva behind end of tube. Tube is 3 to 4 mm longer than essential, as can be seen at its nasal end. (Longer tube was used to allow better view.)

This method is not more difficult than the use of nasal flap alone, and with it one can be less concerned about tension on the flap. It is important to place raw surface against raw surface and to have epithelium placed where it will line the channel. The epithelial surface is not easily recognized with conjunctival flaps. I prefer to leave the Pyrex tube in place for a few months or longer if the patient has no symptoms.

The use of lacrimal sac mucosa in the rare case of congenitally enlarged sacs with obstructions at both ends seems to have merit in the limited number of cases in which it has been used.

Conjunctivodacryocystostomy. Stallard[4] devised an operation to relieve epiphora in patients who had stenosed canaliculi but patent lacrimal sacs and nasolacrimal ducts. As with other types of reconstructive surgery, many of the anastomoses will function satisfactorily. In others the new opening created by cutting off the dome of the sac may tend to close.

The incision is begun about 3 to 4 mm above the medial palpebral tendon and carried inferiorly in a nearly straight line down through the periosteum for a distance of about 20 mm, thus severing the tendon. The lacrimal sac is freed from its dome, where it is tightly bound, to the beginning of the nasolacrimal duct by dissection from the surrounding tissues. A suture is placed through the dome of the sac. The caruncle is excised. A stab incision is passed from the lacus lacrimalis into the lacrimal sac region, a distance of about 5 mm. Manipulation

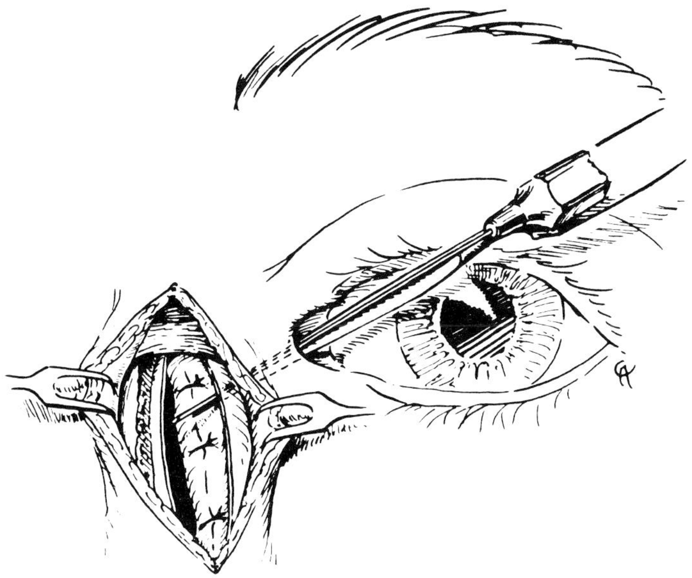

Fig. 10-15. Conjunctivodacryocystorhinostomy. Graefe knife inserted behind guide needle. Knife and needle enter lacrimal sac just posteriorly to anterior flap of sac. Posterior nasal mucosal and lacrimal sac flaps have been sutured together. (From Jones, L. T.: Arch Ophthalmol **66**:111-124, 1961. Copyright 1961, American Medical Association.)

of a small curved hemostat easily enlarges this channel. The hemostat is then used to grasp the suture previously passed through the dome of the sac to pull the dome through the new channel into the caruncle region. Four sutures are inserted into the wall of the sac near its dome. These sutures are then tied to the conjunctiva. The dome of the sac is then cut off.

I prefer to use a Pyrex tube about 4 to 5 mm in length and flanged on the canthal end, as shown in Fig. 10-12. The Pyrex tube can be inserted into the new sac opening to extend 4 to 5 mm down into the sac. The tendency is to insert a tube that is too long. The tube is anchored in its proper position by passing a Dacron suture through the small hole in its flanged end made for that purpose. The Pyrex tube usually can be removed permanently after a few months or left in indefinitely if tear drainage is adequate and irritation is negligible.

Stallard made a vertical incision into the orbital fascia behind the lacrimal sac to let orbital fat herniate into the lacrimal fossa. I prefer to remove the bone that is normally removed when doing an external dacryocystorhinostomy as well as the exposed nasal mucosa. An alternative to removing the nasal mucosa is to incise the nasal mucosa in a U-shaped flap hinged superiorly. The raw surfaces of this flap can be sutured together. If the original procedure is not successful, a Pyrex tube can be inserted as an office procedure without making a skin incision.

Jones[1] described a technique for performing a conjunctivodacryocystorhinostomy (Figs. 10-15 and 10-16). There is no question that many patients will

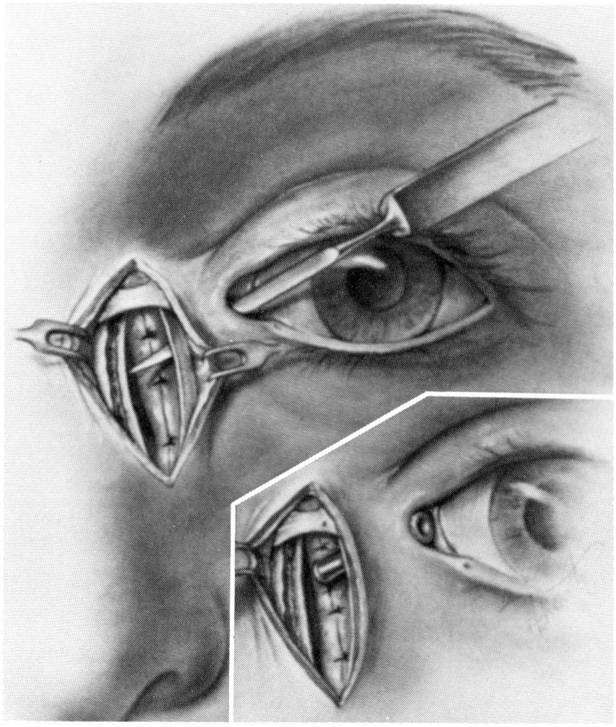

Fig. 10-16. Conjunctivodacryocystorhinostomy. Needle has been removed. Inset shows Pyrex tube in place. (From Jones, L. T.: Arch Ophthalmol 66:111-124, 1961. Copyright 1961, American Medical Association.)

obtain gratifying results when this procedure is performed correctly. I have performed this technique many times. As with all other operations to get the tears to drain properly, there can be complications. The Pyrex tube drains tears better than does the plastic tube in my experience. All types of tubes left in newly created channels may have a propensity to migrate either outward or too far inward. Even with use of a Dacron suture to anchor the tube in proper position, in time the tube will occasionally get out of its proper position.

The nasal end of the Pyrex tube must be properly positioned. If this end hits the tissue of the middle turbinate, the tip of the turbinate may be easily removed with a cupped ethmoid biting forceps. This is usually done at the time of the original operation but can be done later by the intranasal route if necessary.

If the tube is too long, it may lie against the nasal septum and not drain, even if the nasal end is slanted; if the tube is too short, fluid cannot enter the nose. The tip of the Pyrex tube can be exceedingly difficult to visualize within the nose because it is clear. Manufacturers will gold-tip the nasal end of the tubes if requested, which helps in locating them.

Replacing the Pyrex tube after removal for cleansing or other reasons is not always easy. If a straight wire about the size of a no. 2 or 3 Bowman probe is

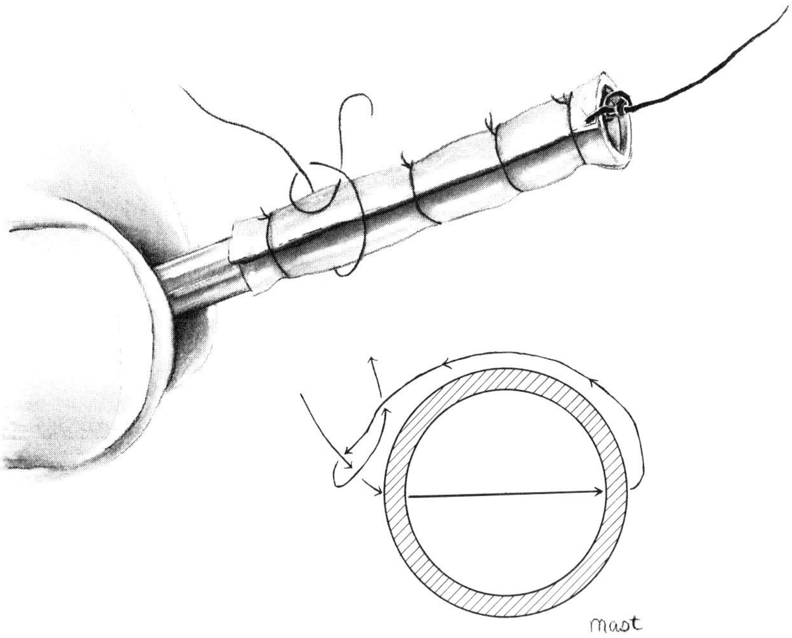

Fig. 10-17. Extremely thin skin graft wrapped, raw surface outward, over 3-mm (outside diameter) silicone tube. Graft is sutured in place with 6-0 silk passed through graft and tube and then wrapped around it. The 5-0 silk suture at end of graft is used to pull tube with graft upward from nose to lacus lacrimalis and to anchor it in position. Tube and graft are left in newly created channel for 2 to 3 weeks to allow graft to take.

threaded into the lumen before the tube is removed, the tube can be guided back over the wire left in the channel.

Use of free grafts

The technique of using free grafts of skin, conjunctiva, or mucosa is somewhat tedious but the long-term functional results can be most gratifying.

The procedure begins as with an external dacryocystorhinostomy except that the lacrimal sac is not utilized. After a large segment of bone is removed to expose the nasal mucosa, as in a dacryocystorhinostomy, the exposed nasal mucosa is excised or flaps are made and sutured in such a manner that the mucosal opening will not close. The caruncle is removed, and a new channel is made from the lacus lacrimalis by directing a sharp instrument medially and slightly downward until the large opening can be seen from the nose. Manipulation of a curved hemostat enlarges this new channel.

Skin is the easiest tissue to use as a free graft. A very thin graft should be taken from the inner surface of the arm with a dermatome such as the Castroviejo. The free skin graft is wrapped around a silicone tube whose outside diameter is 3 mm. The raw surface must be outward and all of the part of the tube

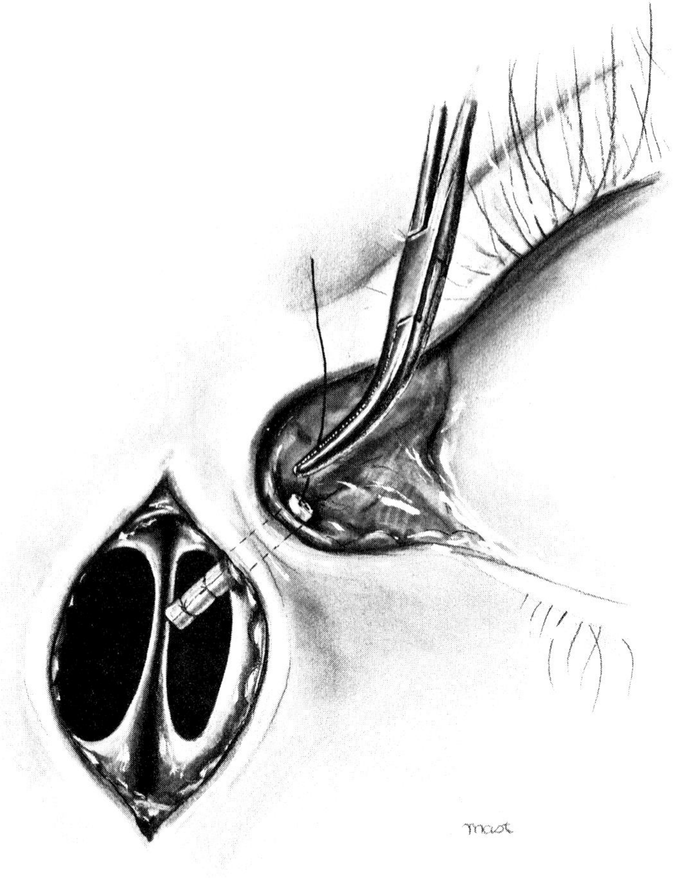

Fig. 10-18. Silicone tube with encircling thin skin graft is pulled from nasal opening into newly created channel by silk suture tied to eye end. Needle will be threaded onto end suture and a bite taken in tissues at lacrimal lake region to anchor tube and graft in position.

that will be used must be covered with the graft. A little overlap of the graft is necessary.

A 6-0 silk suture with an attached sharp needle is run into the middle of the tube (including the graft) and pulled through the opposite side. The suture encircles the graft and is tied to ensure that the graft will not slip on the tube (Fig. 10-17). Usually, about four of these encircling sutures are required. If an assistant holds the silicone tube below the part to be covered and the operator gently holds the graft while the sutures are being placed, this part of the operation will be expedited.

A larger silk suture is placed at the graft end of the tube and knotted tightly. This suture will be used to pull the graft upward through the nostril into the previously created channel to the site from which the caruncle was removed

(Fig. 10-18). It is almost impossible to push the tube from the eye end into the new channel.

Excess at the nasal end of the tube can be cut to the proper length through the original incision. The eye end of the graft is anchored into position by passing a free needle onto the suture and then taking a bite into adjacent soft tissues and tying a knot. After 2 to 3 weeks the silicone tube is removed. By that time the skin graft should have taken, and the new channel should be lined with epithelium. A Pyrex tube of the proper size can be used to replace the silicone tube and left in place as long as desired, usually a matter of weeks, but it can be left in indefinitely if functioning well. Most channels will stay open without the use of the Pyrex tube.

Upper bulbar conjunctiva can be used by ballooning out that conjunctiva with lidocaine and a 30-gauge needle. The conjunctiva is much more difficult to work with than skin. Also, it is often difficult to recognize which side is epithelium and which side is raw surface.

REFERENCES

1. Jones, L. T.: The cure of epiphora due to canalicular disorders, trauma and surgical failures on the lacrimal passages, Trans Am Acad Ophthalmol Otolaryngol 66:506-524, 1962.
2. Morrison, F. D.: An aid to repair of lacerated tear ducts, Arch Ophthalmol 72:341-342, 1964.
3. Schjelderup, H.: Impaired lachrymal drainage, Scand J Plast Reconstr Surg 1-2:30-32, 1967-1968.
4. Stallard, H. B.: Operation for epiphora, Lancet 2:743-744, 1940.
5. Veirs, E. R.: Malleable rods for immediate repair of the traumatically severed lacrimal canaliculus, Trans Am Acad Ophthalmol Otolaryngol 66:263-264, 1962.
6. Worst, J. G. F.: Method for reconstructing torn lacrimal canaliculus, Am J Ophthalmol 53: 520-522, 1962.

CHAPTER 11

Lacrimal gland disorders

ANATOMY OF LACRIMAL GLAND

The lacrimal gland, a rather large tubuloracemose gland, consists of a larger orbital (superior) part and a smaller palpebral (inferior) part separated by the lateral extension of the aponeurosis of the levator palpebrae superioris. The two lobes of the lacrimal gland are connected by lacrimal gland tissue. Indeed, the ductules of the orbital lobe pass through or are adjacent to the palpebral lobe. The lobulated appearance of the gland is an important feature for distinguishing gland from tumor during operation.

Henderson[3] stressed the fact that the gland extends posteriorly almost to the zygomatic sphenoid suture. The blood supply is from the lacrimal branch of the ophthalmic artery; the lacrimal nerve, a branch of the ophthalmic nerve, provides the nerve supply.

The orbital lobe is the main lobe and lies within the orbit in the lacrimal gland fossa, a concavity in the bone in the anterosuperior portion of the orbit. The palpebral lobe of the gland is about one third the size of the orbital portion and lies just beneath the palpebral conjunctiva in the lateral aspect of the upper fornix. The ducts from both lobules of the gland open via 12 or so small apertures just anteriorly to the lateral two fifths of the superior fornix. One or two ducts may open in the lateral extremity of the lower fornix.

Theoretically, excessive tearing can be relieved by closing the ducts by cautery as they empty into the conjunctival sac. I have found the results of this procedure unpredictable.

TUMORS INVOLVING LACRIMAL GLAND

Incidence

These tumors are relatively rare. Nonneoplastic growths (pseudotumors) make up between one fourth and one half of these tumors. Making the proper diagnosis as early as possible and subsequent adequate treatment may offer the only chance of permanent cure of malignant tumors of the gland.

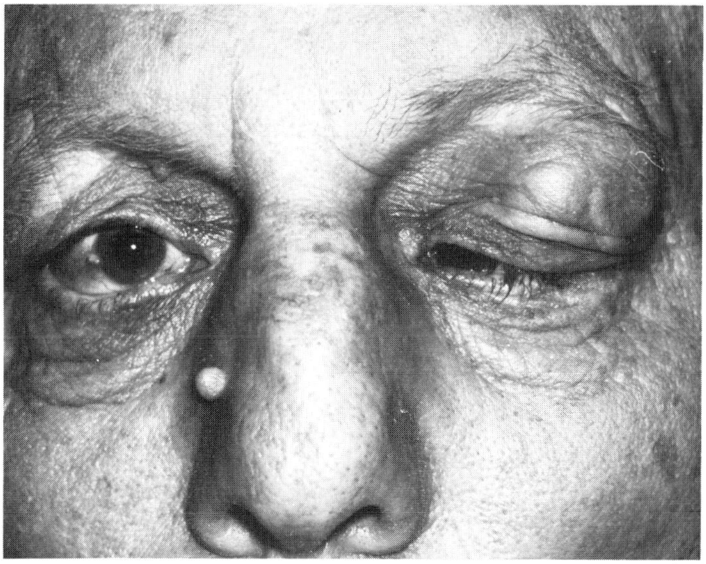

Fig. 11-1. External appearance of patient with mixed tumor of lacrimal gland, showing ptosis, mass in superior temporal position, and eye pushed down and in.

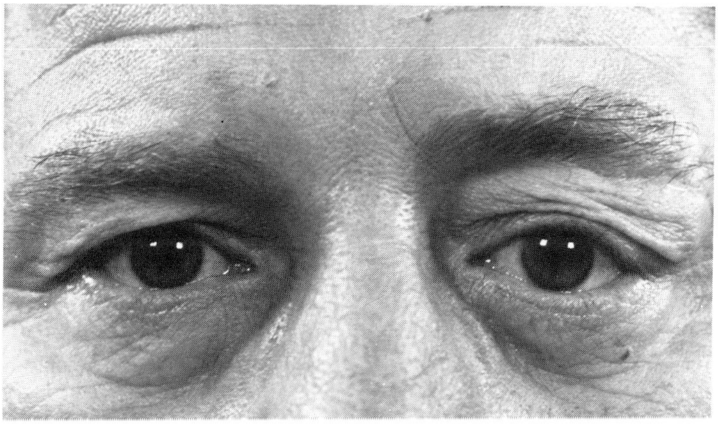

Fig. 11-2. Patient with recurrent mixed cell carcinoma has only minimal swelling of superior temporal region of left orbit with no limitation of eye movements or proptosis. Tumor could be palpated but not with ease.

General appearance

The general appearance may immediately suggest the probability of a tumor of the lacrimal gland (Fig. 11-1). In some patients careful observation is necessary to detect more subtle differences (Fig. 11-2). Swelling of the temporal half of the upper eyelid with ptosis accompanied by displacement of the eye downward and in, as shown in Fig. 11-1, is the classic presentation in malignancies of

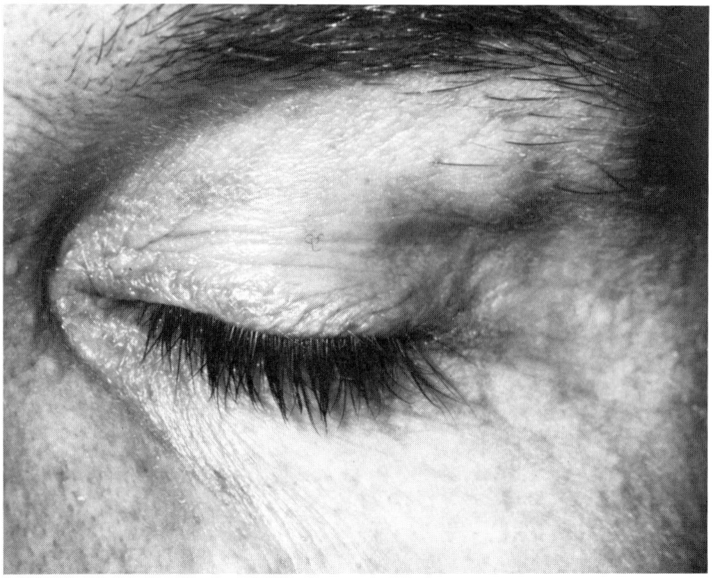

Fig. 11-3. Mild swelling of temporal half of left upper orbital region caused by dermoid cyst in lacrimal gland region. Patient had no functional symptoms. Cyst was large and had been palpable for 4 years or more before swelling and questionable mild ptosis became apparent.

the lacrimal gland, although the degree varies with duration and type of neoplasm. Henderson[3] stressed the importance of the orbital cover test. Gross misalignment of the eyes may be obvious when both eyes are viewed simultaneously from front-face position; however, if right and left orbits are viewed separately by alternately covering the left and the right at the midline of the face, the uncovered eye and adnexal structures may appear normal. Henderson stated that if the eyes look normal when viewed separately, this is diagnostic of slowly growing benign neoplasms and cysts of the orbit, with which the prognosis is favorable.

Palpation of lacrimal gland

In the search for suspected pathologic conditions, primarily tumors, palpation of the lacrimal gland area may be rewarding. Fortunately, one can palpate further posteriorly on the temporal side of the orbit than in other parts. Consequently, a high percentage of tumors in the lacrimal area can be palpated. Tumors of the palpebral lobe of the lacrimal gland are rare but are easily palpated. Dermoid cysts occurring in the lacrimal gland fossa region usually are not difficult to palpate (Fig. 11-3). Malignant tumors of the lacrimal gland may be palpated with some difficulty or with ease, depending on the size of the tumor. The preauricular and cervical glands should be carefully palpated, especially on the ipsilateral side.

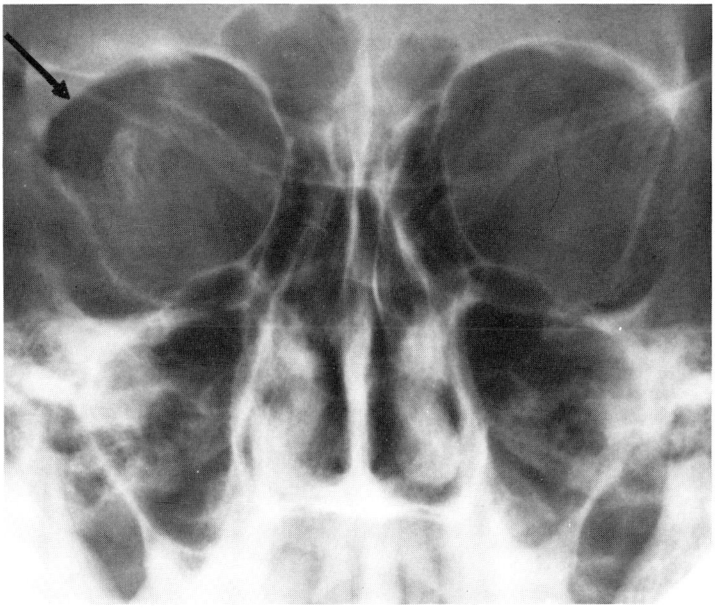

Fig. 11-4. Tomogram of right orbit reveals 2-by-2.5-cm lytic area *(arrow)* in superior lateral wall of orbit with well-defined sclerotic margins. Note calcification in lytic area.

Roentgenologic examination

Roentgenologic examination of the orbit should be performed in every patient suspected of having a tumor involving the lacrimal gland region. There are several roentgenographic findings[6] that suggest tumor of the lacrimal gland:

1. There may be enlargement of the lacrimal fossa with intact bone cortex. A slowly enlarging, expanding mass may cause this and is usually but not always indicative of a benign lesion.

2. There may be increased density of adjacent bone including the superior and lateral orbital rims and the greater wing of the sphenoid. Extensive bone sclerosis may indicate the presence of malignant tumor with bone invasion.

3. There may be extensive erosion and bone destruction. The bone destruction is not always limited to the lacrimal fossa but depends on the direction of tumor growth. Lysis of bone is shown in Fig. 11-4.

Ultrasonography may be of limited help. Computerized axial tomography (EMI scan) can provide evidence of lesions in the vicinity of the lacrimal gland (Fig. 11-5).

General examination

Examination by an internist is advisable for patients suspected of having tumors involving the lacrimal gland. Lymphoma should be ruled out as far as possible. A roentgenogram of the chest should be routine.

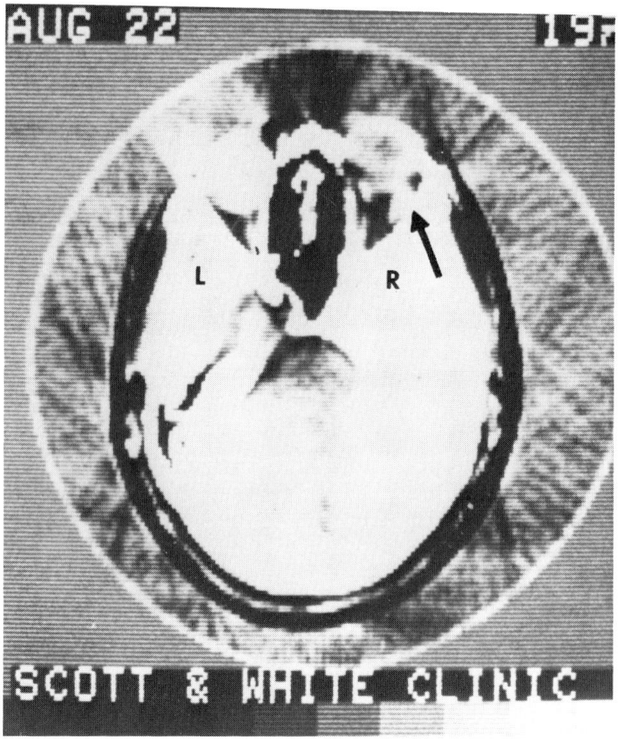

Fig. 11-5. Computerized axial tomography (EMI scan) shows triangular mass in lateral aspect of right retrobulbar space *(arrow)*. This section is above equator. Optic nerve can be seen in medial aspect of each retrobulbar space. Orbital exploration revealed inflammatory pseudotumor.

CLASSIFICATION OF EPITHELIAL TUMORS OF LACRIMAL GLAND

Epithelial tumors of the lacrimal gland are classified according to their histologic features as described by Forrest.[2] His classification is (1) benign and malignant mixed tumors, (2) adenoid cystic carcinomas, and (3) all others. Another commonly used classification is (1) mixed tumors, benign or malignant, (2) adenoid cystic carcinomas, and (3) adenocarcinomatous and mucoepidermoid carcinomas.

Mixed tumors

Mixed tumors of the lacrimal gland represent more than one half of the epithelial tumors of the lacrimal gland fossa. A disturbing feature of clinically and histologically benign mixed tumors is their propensity to recur and take on malignant characteristics. The assumption is that the tumor undergoes malignant metaplasia or that small foci of malignant tissue existed but were overlooked in the original histologic examination. Possibly the belief of some pathologists that

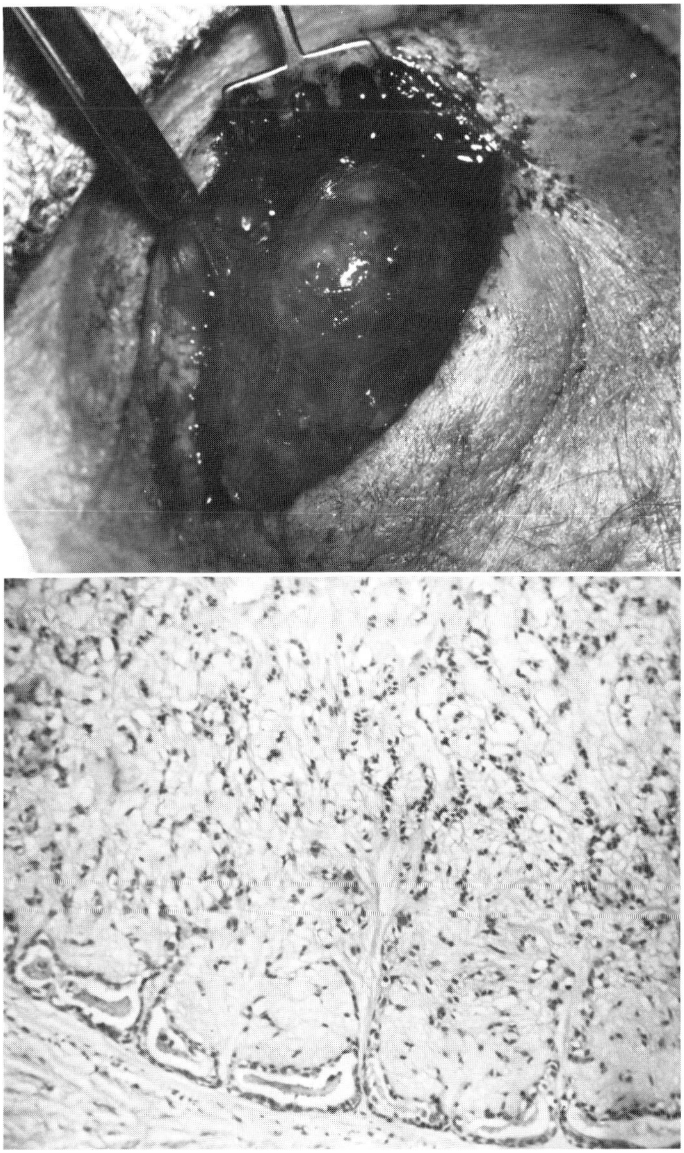

Fig. 11-6. Mixed tumor of lacrimal gland. *Top,* At operation, tumor within its capsule is being carefully dissected out. Tumor was lobulated in outline and had a dense fibrous capsule. *Bottom,* Histologic section shows cords of small uniform epithelial cells set in myxoid stroma. (Hematoxylin and eosin; ×450.)

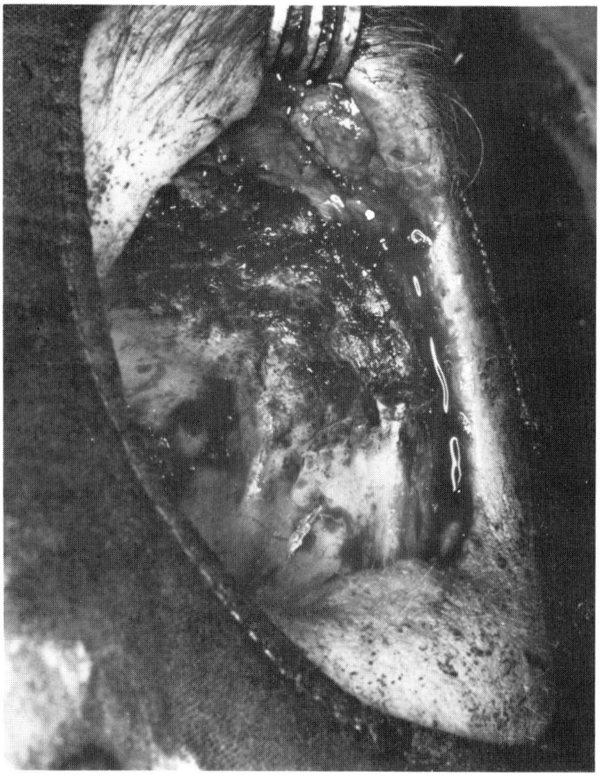

Fig. 11-7. Recurrent mixed cell carcinoma with bone invasion. Treatment included exenteration of orbit, removal of all apparent invaded bone, and thorough cauterization of bone and soft tissue in area where tumor was.

all mixed tumors of the lacrimal gland are malignant is correct. The cure rate is high because of the low grade of malignancy and the encapsulation (unless the tumor outgrows it) (Fig. 11-6). Benign mixed tumors tend to grow slowly. Roentgenograms may show evidence of increased bone density or enlargement of the lacrimal fossa. Tomograms are often revealing. Bone invasion carries a poor diagnosis (Fig. 11-7).

The most characteristic sign of a tumor of the lacrimal gland is the downward and often nasal displacement of the eye and proptosis. Ptosis and fullness of the outer portion of the upper lid will develop as the tumor enlarges. If, in addition, a mass can be palpated in the upper temporal portion of the eye, exploration must be carried out. The biopsy findings determine the further course of action.

In preference to a brow incision (Fig. 11-8) Jones[5] recommended performing biopsy on the gland from the lateral canthal approach (Fig. 11-9). The canthus and ligament are divided horizontally. The ligament holding the upper lid is cut, and the soft tissues are reflected. This brings the inferior lateral portion of the gland into the field for viewing and palpation. A biopsy specimen is taken,

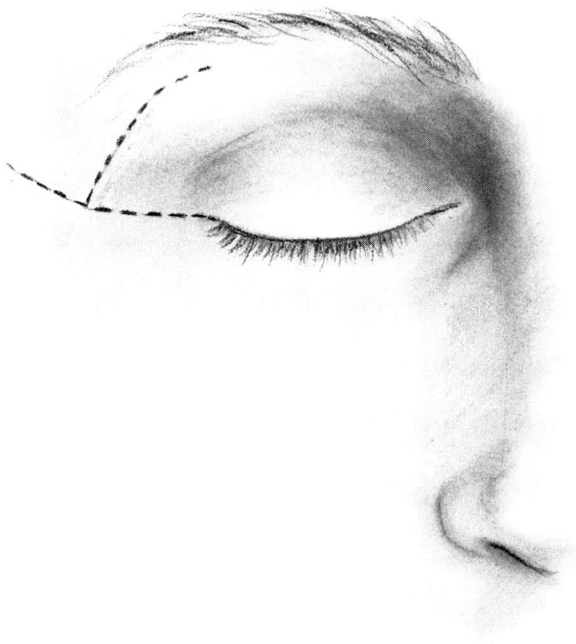

Fig. 11-8. Incision only in brow is used for direct surgical approach to lacrimal gland. Posterior and lateral extension of gland can be missed with this incision. (Redrawn after Jones, I. S.: South Med J **64**:1503-1504, 1971.)

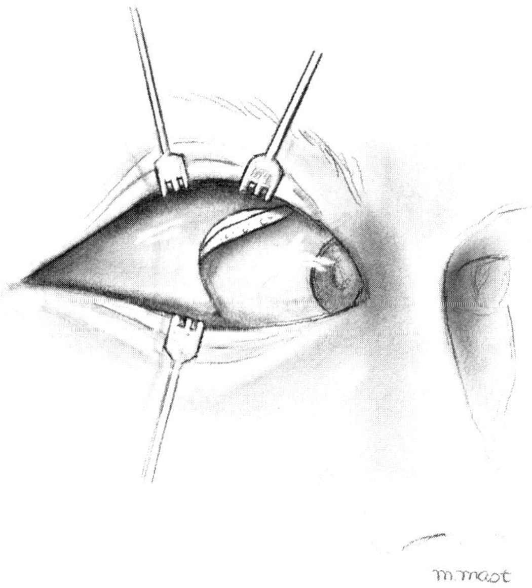

Fig. 11-9. Lateral canthotomy approach to lacrimal gland. Canthus and ligament are divided horizontally. Ligament holding upper lid is cut, and soft tissue is retracted, exposing inferior lateral portion of gland. (Redrawn after Jones, I. S.: South Med J **64**:1503-1504, 1971.)

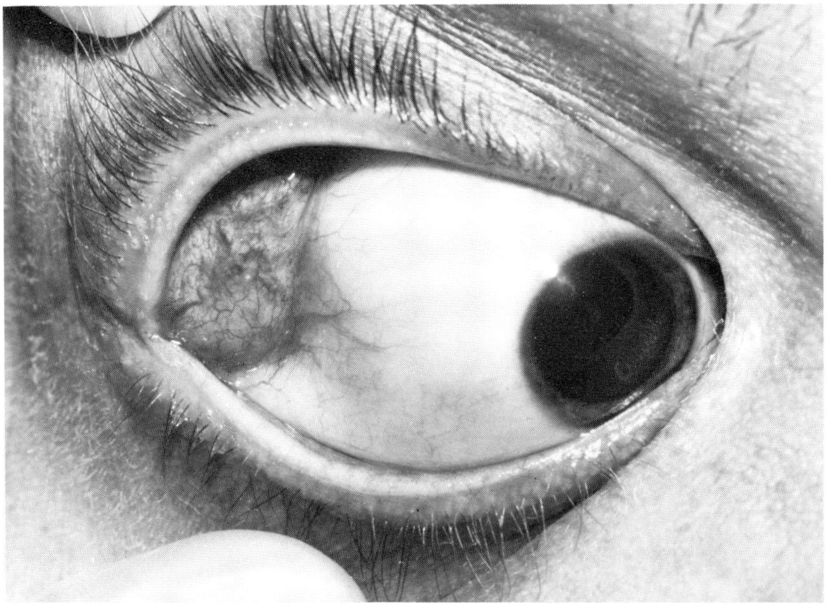

Fig. 11-10. Adenoid cystic carcinoma. Patient lived more than 3 years after exenteration; death was from vascular disease.

and the wound is easily closed. This same route is used if excision of the gland and bone proves necessary.

If a benign mixed tumor is diagnosed, the treatment is careful excision in toto, with care to avoid rupturing the capsule; the same approach is used for dermoids.

Adenoid cystic carcinoma

Adenoid carcinoma is the most common epithelial malignancy of the lacrimal gland. The prognosis is grave compared to that of mixed tumors of the gland. Hogan and Zimmerman[1] stressed the importance of recognizing this difference. The adenoid cystic carcinoma is highly malignant with early invasion of local bone and soft tissues (Fig. 11-10). Metastasis to other parts of the body is common. Radical operation is the only chance for cure. If biopsy shows this type of tumor, the surgeon should be prepared for immediate exenteration of the orbit, including the eyelids. Because bone invasion occurs early, as much of the bone of the lacrimal fossa region as is feasible should be removed. In addition, this region, including bone and adjacent soft tissue margins, should be vigorously cauterized with a ball-point cautery.

Treatment of malignancies of lacrimal gland

Postoperative irradiation may be given in cases of high-grade malignancy, especially if there is doubt about all the tumor being removed. In general, how-

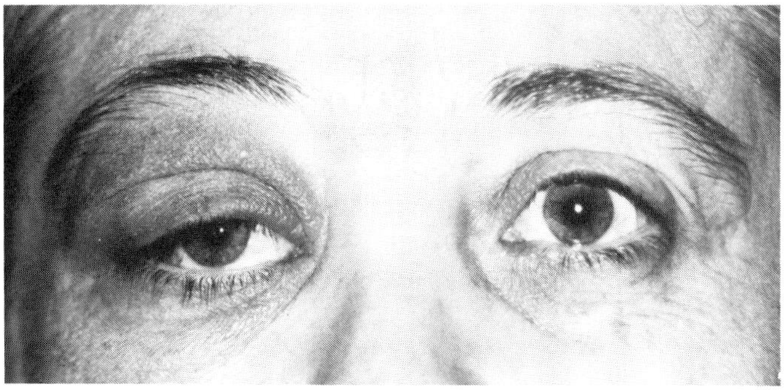

Fig. 11-11. Lymphoid pseudotumor. About 1 year prior to date of picture, patient noticed lump in right upper eyelid and that right eye was becoming more prominent than left. Ptosis is present, and tumorlike mass was palpable in right lacrimal gland region extending well back into orbit.

ever, irradiation is not thought to be very effective against lacrimal gland malignancies. Finally, the patient should be instructed to return for routine reexamination at appropriate intervals or sooner if there is any sign of recurrence.

Lymphomas should be treated under the supervision of cancer specialists.

Other disorders of the lacrimal gland

Pseudotumors. Clinically, pseudotumors cannot be distinguished from neoplastic tumors. They occur fairly commonly within the orbit. When Blodi and Gass[1] biopsied 140 orbits of patients with pseudotumors, they found that the lacrimal gland often was affected, markedly so in nine cases. The pseudotumors fall into two general classifications:

1. Inflammatory pseudotumor. This may represent the advanced stage of a chronic dacryoadenitis. Histologically, the normal secretory cells of the gland and ducts are destroyed and are replaced by connective tissue and inflammatory cells.

2. Lymphoid pseudotumor. This tumor (Fig. 11-11) also has been called "reactive lymphoid hyperplasia." There is marked infiltration of lymphoid cells, plasma cells, and reticulum cells (Fig. 11-12). The critical problem is differentiation of malignant lymphoma from reactive lymphoid hyperplasia. Hogan and Zimmerman[4] pointed out the characteristics that indicate that the reactive lymphoid pseudotumor is benign: polymorphism and the admixture of polymorphonuclear leukocytes, eosinophils, plasma cells, and macrophages. These features suggest inflammatory rather than malignant disease. Treatment is usually not indicated. The gland can be excised if necessary.

Tumors simulating lacrimal gland tumors

There are many tumors that simulate lacrimal gland tumors, and the diagnosis may have to rest on histologic evidence. Fig. 11-13 shows some tumors that

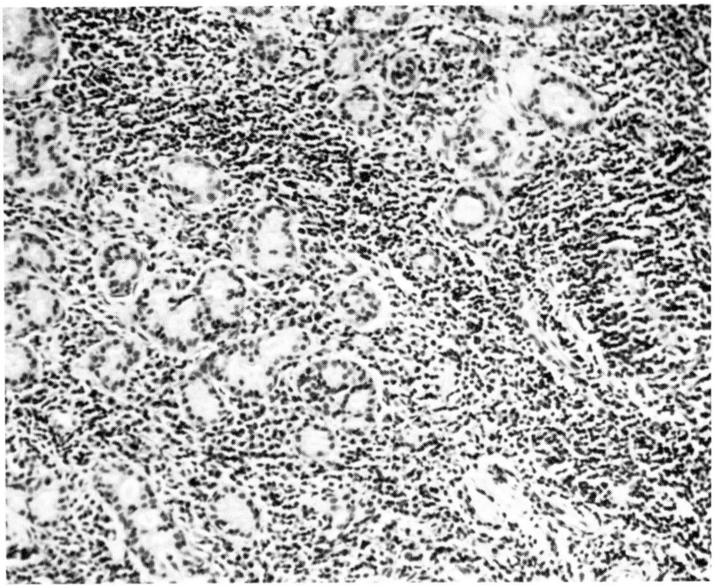

Fig. 11-12. Histologic features of lymphoid pseudotumor, showing dense inflammatory infiltrate composed predominantly of lymphocytes within lacrimal gland. (Hematoxylin and eosin; ×450.)

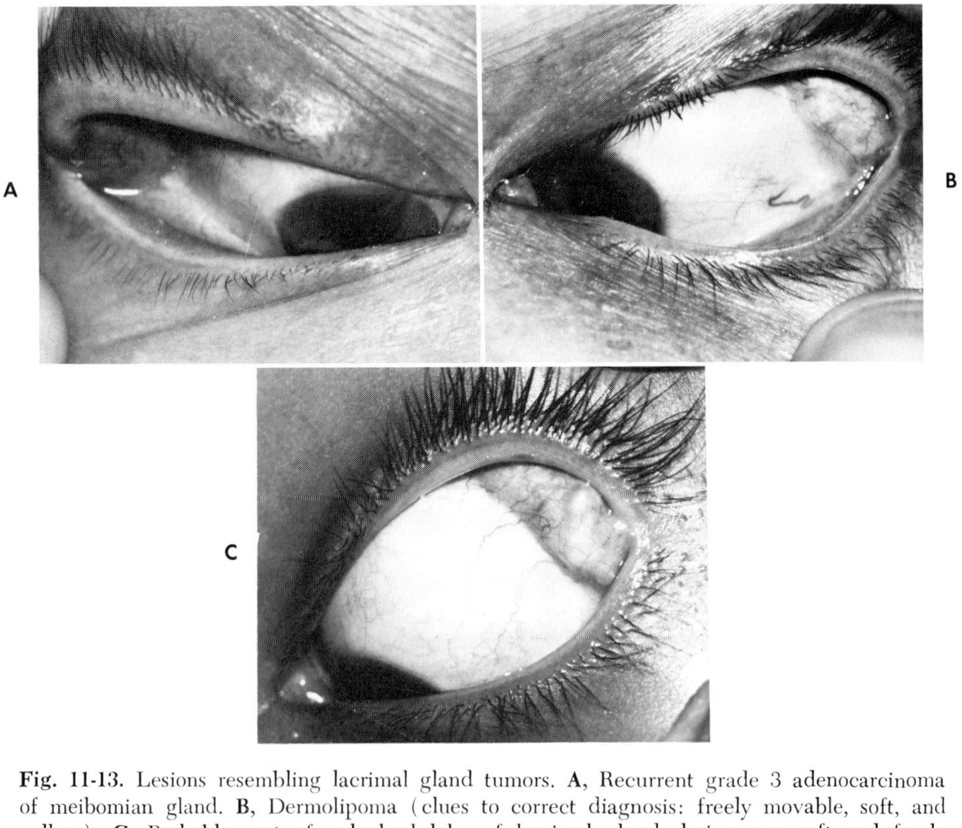

Fig. 11-13. Lesions resembling lacrimal gland tumors. **A,** Recurrent grade 3 adenocarcinoma of meibomian gland. **B,** Dermolipoma (clues to correct diagnosis: freely movable, soft, and yellow). **C,** Probable cyst of palpebral lobe of lacrimal gland; lesion was soft and freely movable. Observation is indicated.

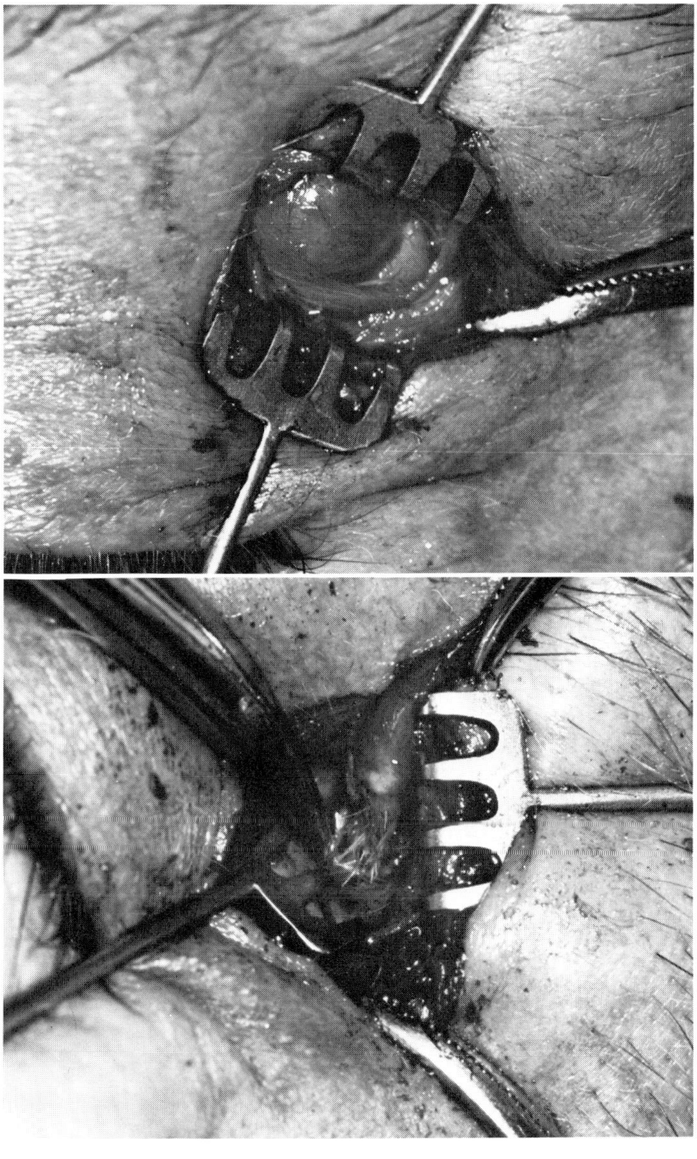

Fig. 11-14. Dermoid cyst in lacrimal gland region. *Top,* Capsule is in view. Temporal bony margin is easily seen. Swelling had been gradually increasing for about 4 years. *Bottom,* After rupture of cyst, hair is visible within it. Cyst extended deeply into orbit.

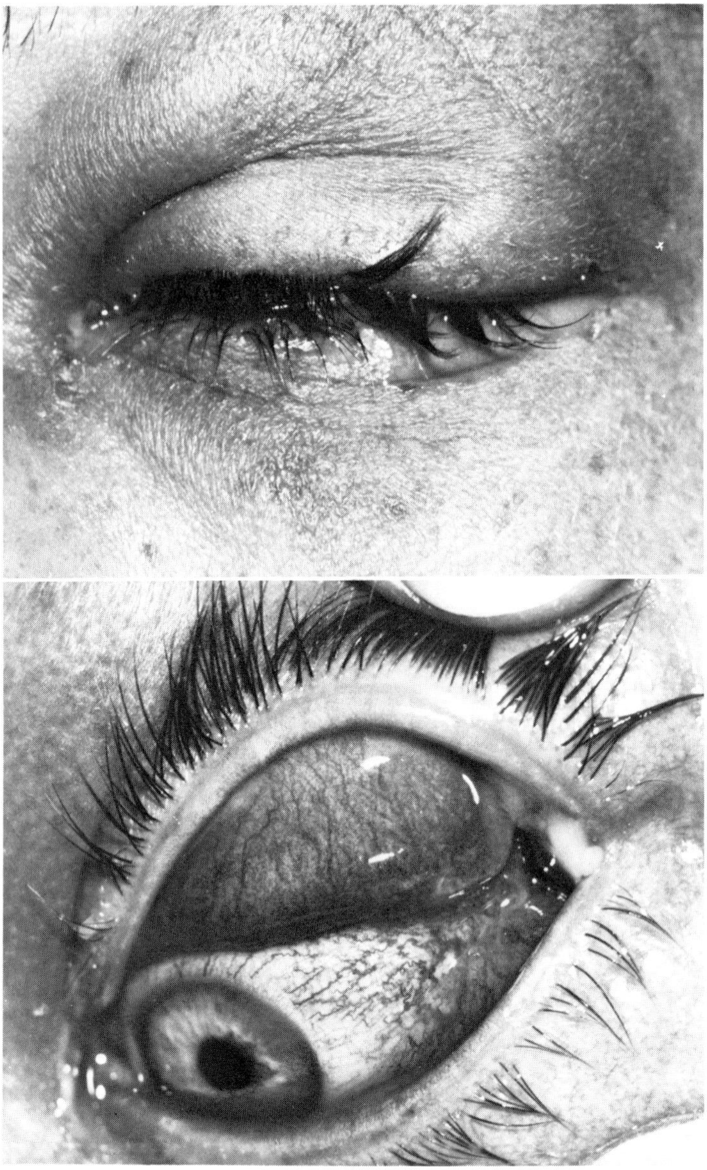

Fig. 11-15. Acute suppurative dacryoadenitis. *Top,* Edematous lid with ptosis, pain, and lacrimation. *Bottom,* At later date, less edema and more purulent discharge.

cannot be distinguished from serious lacrimal gland neoplasm by external appearance alone.

Dermoid cysts. Dermoid cysts (Fig. 11-14) in the lacrimal gland region are very uncommon and slow to enlarge. The lesion can be palpated in the lacrimal gland region, but the diagnosis cannot be established except by excision. There is no reliable method of determining preoperatively how far posteriorly they ex-

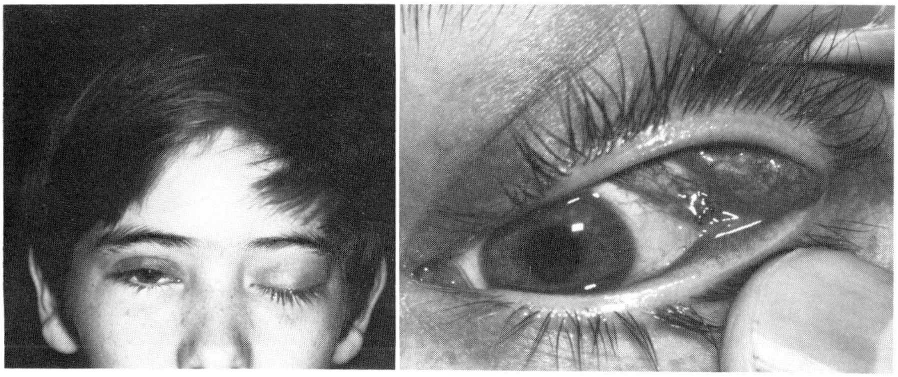

Fig. 11-16. Acute dacryoadenitis of possible viral origin. *Left,* At 2 weeks before picture taken, sudden onset of bilateral acute dacryocystitis with edema, hyperemia, fever, and excess tearing. At time of picture, right eye markedly improved; left eye had developed ptosis and limitation of vertical movement. *Right,* Enlarged hyperemic lacrimal gland on left side. There was minimal evidence of inflammation 3 weeks after onset.

tend; it can be a considerable distance. Their removal presents problems. Those extending far back into the orbit require removal of bone laterally. When possible, a less radical procedure to remove the cyst without breaking the capsule is preferable.

Acute dacryoadenitis. Acute dacryoadenitis is caused by a wide variety of diseases such as measles, herpes simplex, pneumonia, influenza, and herpes zoster. Acute suppurative dacryoadenitis (Fig. 11-15) is rare and is caused by several kinds of bacteria. Acute dacryoadenitis without suppuration (Fig. 11-16) may be viral in origin.

Chronic dacryoadenitis. Chronic dacryoadenitis is rare. Sarcoidosis is perhaps most frequently implicated. Syphilis, tuberculosis, and trachoma also may cause a chronic dacryoadenitis.

Treatment is usually that of the general condition associated with the lacrimal gland inflammation.

REFERENCES

1. Blodi, F. C., and Gass, J. D.: Inflammatory pseudotumor of the orbit, Trans Am Acad Ophthalmol Otolaryngol 71:303-323, 1967.
2. Forrest, A. W.: Epithelial tumors of the lacrimal gland. In Veirs, E. R., editor: The lacrimal system, Proceedings of the first international symposium, St. Louis, 1971, The C. V. Mosby Co., pp. 19-28.
3. Henderson, J. W.: Orbital tumors, Philadelphia, 1973, W. B. Saunders Company.
4. Hogan, M. J., and Zimmerman, L. E.: Ophthalmic pathology, ed. 2, Philadelphia, 1962, W. B. Saunders Company.
5. Jones, I. S.: Tumors of the lacrimal glands: their surgical management, South Med J 64: 1503-1504, 1971.
6. Newton, T. H.: Roentgen appearance of lacrimal-gland tumors, Radiology 79:598-605, 1962.

Index